Virulence Factors and Antibiotic Resistance of Enterobacterales

Virulence Factors and Antibiotic Resistance of Enterobacterales

Editors

Dobroslava Bujňáková
Nikola Puvača
Ivana Ćirković

MDPI • Basel • Beijing • Wuhan • Barcelona • Belgrade • Manchester • Tokyo • Cluj • Tianjin

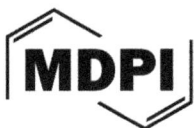

Editors

Dobroslava Bujňáková
Department of Digestive Tract Physiology
Center of Biosciences of the Slovak Academy of Sciences
Košice
Slovakia

Nikola Puvača
Department of Engineering Management in Biotechnology
University BA in Novi Sad
Novi Sad
Serbia

Ivana Ćirković
Institute of Microbiology and Immunology,
Faculty of Medicine
University of Belgrade
Belgrade
Serbia

Editorial Office
MDPI
St. Alban-Anlage 66
4052 Basel, Switzerland

This is a reprint of articles from the Special Issue published online in the open access journal *Microorganisms* (ISSN 2076-2607) (available at: www.mdpi.com/journal/microorganisms/special_issues/antibiotic_Enterobacterales).

For citation purposes, cite each article independently as indicated on the article page online and as indicated below:

LastName, A.A.; LastName, B.B.; LastName, C.C. Article Title. *Journal Name* **Year**, *Volume Number*, Page Range.

ISBN 978-3-0365-2781-9 (Hbk)
ISBN 978-3-0365-2780-2 (PDF)

© 2021 by the authors. Articles in this book are Open Access and distributed under the Creative Commons Attribution (CC BY) license, which allows users to download, copy and build upon published articles, as long as the author and publisher are properly credited, which ensures maximum dissemination and a wider impact of our publications.

The book as a whole is distributed by MDPI under the terms and conditions of the Creative Commons license CC BY-NC-ND.

Contents

About the Editors vii

Preface to "Virulence Factors and Antibiotic Resistance of Enterobacterales" ix

Momen Askoura, Ahmad J. Almalki, Amr S. Abu Lila, Khaled Almansour, Farhan Alshammari, El-Sayed Khafagy, Tarek S. Ibrahim and Wael A. H. Hegazy
Alteration of *Salmonella enterica* Virulence and Host Pathogenesis through Targeting *sdiA* by Using the CRISPR-Cas9 System
Reprinted from: *Microorganisms* **2021**, *9*, 2564, doi:10.3390/microorganisms9122564 1

Manuel G. Ballesteros-Monrreal, Margarita M. P. Arenas-Hernández, Edwin Barrios-Villa, Josue Juarez, Maritza Lizeth Álvarez-Ainza, Pablo Taboada, Rafael De la Rosa-López, Enrique Bolado-Martínez and Dora Valencia
Bacterial Morphotypes as Important Trait for Uropathogenic *E. coli* Diagnostic; a Virulence-Phenotype-Phylogeny Study
Reprinted from: *Microorganisms* **2021**, *9*, 2381, doi:10.3390/microorganisms9112381 19

Marta Gómez, Arancha Valverde, Rosa del Campo, Juan Miguel Rodríguez and Antonio Maldonado-Barragán
Phenotypic and Molecular Characterization of Commensal, Community-Acquired and Nosocomial *Klebsiella* spp.
Reprinted from: *Microorganisms* **2021**, *9*, 2344, doi:10.3390/microorganisms9112344 41

Jianxin Gao, Zhonghui Han, Ping Li, Hongyan Zhang, Xinjun Du and Shuo Wang
Outer Membrane Protein F Is Involved in Biofilm Formation, Virulence and Antibiotic Resistance in *Cronobacter sakazakii*
Reprinted from: *Microorganisms* **2021**, *9*, 2338, doi:10.3390/microorganisms9112338 59

Maelys Proquot, Lovasoa Najaraly Jamal, Chloe Plouzeau-Jayle, Anthony Michaud, Lauranne Broutin, Christophe Burucoa, Julie Cremniter and Maxime Pichon
K1 Antigen Is Associated with Different AST Profile in *Escherichia coli*: A One-Month-Long Pilot Study
Reprinted from: *Microorganisms* **2021**, *9*, 1884, doi:10.3390/microorganisms9091884 73

Dobroslava Bujňáková, Lívia Karahutová and Vladimír Kmeť
Escherichia coli Specific Virulence-Gene Markers Analysis for Quality Control of Ovine Cheese in Slovakia
Reprinted from: *Microorganisms* **2021**, *9*, 1808, doi:10.3390/microorganisms9091808 83

Racha Beyrouthy, Carolina Sabença, Frédéric Robin, Patricia Poeta, Giberto Igrejas and Richard Bonnet
Successful Dissemination of Plasmid-Mediated Extended-Spectrum β-Lactamases in Enterobacterales over Humans to Wild Fauna
Reprinted from: *Microorganisms* **2021**, *9*, 1471, doi:10.3390/microorganisms9071471 95

Lívia Karahutová, René Mandelík and Dobroslava Bujňáková
Antibiotic Resistant and Biofilm-Associated *Escherichia coli* Isolates from Diarrheic and Healthy Dogs
Reprinted from: *Microorganisms* **2021**, *9*, 1334, doi:10.3390/microorganisms9061334 107

About the Editors

Dobroslava Bujňáková

Dobroslava Bujňáková is a scientific researcher and head of the Laboratory of Microbial Genetic at the Department of Digestive Tract Physiology at the Institute of Animal Physiology, Centre of Biosciences of the Slovak Academy of Sciences in Košice, Slovakia.

She is a microbiologist with experience in the field of animal microflora of the digestive tract, Maldi Tof diagnostics of bacteria, PCR diagnostics of virulence, "fitness" factors, and antibiotic resistance.

The focus of her research in recent years is lactic acid bacteria with regard to the qualified assessment of their safety-QPS, functionality, and their technological properties; natural alternatives to antibiotics; evaluation of antibiotic resistance and virulence in Enterobacterales in foods and animals; and the study of molecular analysis of bacterial biofilm and communication, quorum sensing. She was the principal investigator and co-solver of several national and international projects concerning to mentioned issues.

Dobroslava is serving as a guest editor and peer reviewer for several indexed journals. Her citation index is 14. She has been a mentor of PhD dissertations, bachelor and master theses and she also provides practical and theoretical lectures at the University of Veterinary Medicine and Pharmacy in Košice within the study subject Biochemistry.

Nikola Puvača

Nikola Puvača is an Associate Professor at the Department of Engineering Management in Biotechnology of the University Business Academy in Novi Sad, Serbia. He is a multidisciplinary scientist with Ph.D. diplomas in Biotechnology, Veterinary Medicine, and Human Medicine, and a postdoctoral diploma in Toxicology and Molecular Genetics. He has significant experience in animal and poultry science, with a major interest in nutrition, feed quality and safety, natural alternatives for antibiotics, and antimicrobial resistance. He is involved in many research collaborations in various science fields. He is serving as an Editorial Board Member and peer reviewer for many indexed journals, and he is the author of more than 200 scientific papers published in international journals and the proceedings of national and international conferences. He is a guest lecturer in several international universities and has won many rewards for scientific and professional work. Currently, he is in the position of Vice Dean for Internarial Relations at his home faculty.

Ivana Ćirković

Ivana Ćirković, MD, PhD, is a Full Professor at the University of Belgrade–Faculty of Medicine, Belgrade, Serbia, a specialist in Microbiology and subspecialist in Clinical Microbiology, with more than 10 years of postdoctoral experience and 19 years of experience in the field of clinical and experimental microbiology, particularly focusing on the genotypic and phenotypic characterization of antibiotic-resistant bacteria, with a strong publication record in peer-reviewed journals (citations: 1376; h-index: 13). She has documented experience in successfully materializing multidisciplinary projects in Serbia and internationally. Additionally, Ivana Ćirković is an ECDC National Microbiology Focal Point and member of the General Committee of European Committee of Antimicrobial Susceptibility Testing (EUCAST). Notably, Ivana Ćirković has obtained substantial leadership and organizational skills by ensuring the smooth and efficient running of the National Reference Laboratory of Staphylococcus and Enterococcus at the Institute of Microbiology and Immunology, and believing that imparting knowledge to new generations of scientists is of utmost importance, she has also been a mentor of six PhD dissertations and numerous bachelor and master theses.

Preface to "Virulence Factors and Antibiotic Resistance of Enterobacterales"

The heterogeneous group of Gram-negative bacteria such as *Escherichia coli* and non-*Escherichia coli* Enterobacterales (e.g., *Klebsiella*, *Enterobacter*, *Citrobacter*) that can colonize the gastrointestinal tract of humans and animals and persist as gut commensals without inducing any infections in the environment with balanced microbiota (colonization resistance) also harbor features responsible for virulence and pathogenicity, including "fitness factors" or phenotypes that may result in severe health concerns, such as biofilm formation and/or multidrug resistance. Pathogenic Enterobacterales isolated from infected patients are the most often investigated, but also fecal isolates from healthy subjects including food, companion, and wild animals and/or food or environmental strains should be a more frequent target, aiming to determine the pathogenic potential of a wider biodiversity reservoir.

This book compiles research on Enterobacterales characterization concerning the presence of genes associated with virulence (adhesins; surface cellulose structures and curli; siderophores, e.g., enterobactin, aerobactin, and yersiniabactin; protectines; invasins or toxins), and, furthermore, bacterial-biofilm-associated phenotypes. Although not directly involved in pathogenicity, the acquisition of multiple antibiotic resistances strongly supports the success of opportunistic Enterobacterales pathogens in invasion, survival, and spread and markedly complicates the treatment of infections. Not only pathogens, but also commensal bacteria, considered harmless and part of the normal microbiota, are exposed to selection pressure and can be a reservoir of mobile genetic elements carrying antibiotic resistance genes. Therefore, the occurrence of drug-resistant bacteria within a commensal population and the possibility to exchange genetic material through horizontal gene transfer may represent a major health concern.

Dobroslava Bujňáková, Nikola Puvača, Ivana Ćirković
Editors

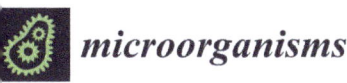

Article

Alteration of *Salmonella enterica* Virulence and Host Pathogenesis through Targeting *sdiA* by Using the CRISPR-Cas9 System

Momen Askoura [1,*], Ahmad J. Almalki [2,3], Amr S. Abu Lila [4,5], Khaled Almansour [5], Farhan Alshammari [5], El-Sayed Khafagy [6,7], Tarek S. Ibrahim [2] and Wael A. H. Hegazy [1,*]

1. Department of Microbiology and Immunology, Faculty of Pharmacy, Zagazig University, Zagazig 44519, Egypt
2. Department of Pharmaceutical Chemistry, Faculty of Pharmacy, King Abdulaziz University, Jeddah 21589, Saudi Arabia; ajalmalki@kau.edu.sa (A.J.A.); tmabrahem@kau.edu.sa (T.S.I.)
3. Center of Excellence for Drug Research and Pharmaceutical Industries, King Abdulaziz University, Jeddah 21589, Saudi Arabia
4. Department of Pharmaceutics and Industrial Pharmacy, Faculty of Pharmacy, Zagazig University, Zagazig 44519, Egypt; a.abulila@uoh.edu.sa
5. Department of Pharmaceutics, College of Pharmacy, University of Hail, Hail 81442, Saudi Arabia; kh.almansour@uoh.edu.sa (K.A.); frh.alshammari@uoh.edu.sa (F.A.)
6. Department of Pharmaceutics, College of Pharmacy, Prince Sattam Bin Abdulaziz University, Al-kharj 11942, Saudi Arabia; e.khafagy@psau.edu.sa
7. Department of Pharmaceutics and Industrial Pharmacy, Faculty of Pharmacy, Suez Canal University, Ismailia 41552, Egypt
* Correspondence: momenaskora@yahoo.com (M.A.); waelmhegazy@daad-alumni.de (W.A.H.H.); Tel.: +20-1125226642 (M.A.); +20-1101188800 (W.A.H.H.)

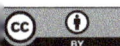

Abstract: *Salmonella enterica* is a common cause of many enteric infections worldwide and is successfully engineered to deliver heterologous antigens to be used as vaccines. Clustered Regularly Interspaced Short Palindromic Repeats (CRISPRs) RNA-guided Cas9 endonuclease is a promising genome editing tool. In the current study, a CRISPR-Cas9 system was used to target *S. enterica sdiA* that encodes signal molecule receptor SdiA and responds to the quorum sensing (QS) signaling compounds N-acylhomoserine lactones (AHLs). For this purpose, *sdiA* was targeted in both *S. enterica* wild type (WT) and the ΔssaV mutant strain, where SsaV has been reported to be an essential component of SPI2-T3SS. The impact of *sdiA* mutation on *S. enterica* virulence was evaluated at both early invasion and later intracellular replication in both the presence and absence of AHL. Additionally, the influence of *sdiA* mutation on the pathogenesis *S. enterica* WT and mutants was investigated in vivo, using mice infection model. Finally, the minimum inhibitory concentrations (MICs) of various antibiotics against *S. enterica* strains were determined. Present findings show that mutation in *sdiA* significantly affects *S. enterica* biofilm formation, cell adhesion and invasion. However, *sdiA* mutation did not affect bacterial intracellular survival. Moreover, in vivo bacterial pathogenesis was markedly lowered in *S. enterica* ΔsdiA in comparison with the wild-type strain. Significantly, double-mutant *sdiA* and *ssaV* attenuated the *S. enterica* virulence and in vivo pathogenesis. Moreover, mutations in selected genes increased *Salmonella* susceptibility to tested antibiotics, as revealed by determining the MICs and MBICs of these antibiotics. Altogether, current results clearly highlight the importance of the CRISPR-Cas9 system as a bacterial genome editing tool and the valuable role of SdiA in *S. enterica* virulence. The present findings extend the understanding of virulence regulation and host pathogenesis of *Salmonella enterica*.

Keywords: *Salmonella enterica*; CRISPR-Cas9; *sdiA*; *ssaV*; virulence; pathogenesis

1. Introduction

Salmonella enterica are facultative anaerobic intracellular Gram-negative non-lactose fermenting motile bacteria that belong to the family Enterobacteriaceae. *S. enterica* infections greatly vary from a mild gastroenteritis, caused mostly by *S. enterica* serovars Typhimurium (*S.* Typhimurium) and Enteritidis (*S.* Enteritidis), to serious systemic infections of typhoid fever caused by *S. enterica* serovar Typhi (*S.* Typhi) or Paratyphi (*S.* Paratyphi) [1]. The encoding genes for numerous significant virulence factors of *S. enterica* are arranged in specific loci called *Salmonella* Pathogenicity Islands (SPI) [2]. *Salmonella* deploys intricate virulence factors named type III secretion systems (TTSS), which mediate distinct functions [3]. Two major SPI encode TTSS to translocate *Salmonella* effectors in different phases of pathogenesis [4]. SPI1-TTSS translocates TTSS effector proteins into host cell cytoplasm during early stages of invasion, while SPI2-TTSS translocates TTSS effector proteins responsible for bacterial intracellular survival at later stages [2,5]. Previous studies described the role of the SPI2-T3SS machinery component SsaV and its importance for the secretion of most T3SS effectors [6–8]. Importantly, mutations in *ssaV* could lead to a significant reduction in *S. enterica* virulence through decreasing the translocation of SPI2-effector proteins, as this decrease affects the ability of *S. enterica* to survive intracellularly [7].

Quorum sensing (QS) is a way that bacteria use autoinducer (AI) molecules, such as N-acylhomoserine lactones (AHLs), for cell-to-cell communication, which plays a crucial role in bacterial virulence [9–11]. It has been shown that *S. enterica* contains at least two types of QS systems, one is induced by acylhomoserine lactone (AHL) and the other is induced by autoinducer-2 (AI-2) [12]. *S. enterica* employs QS to enhance bacterial virulence and pathogenesis through regulation of biofilm formation, virulence factors' production and swarming motility [13,14]. *S. enterica* does not encode an AHL synthase, but it encodes SdiA, a LuxR homolog, which detects AHLs. A variety of AHL molecules with different acyl chain length and substituents at the C-3 position have been reported to mediate QS [15]. SdiA detects solely AHLs produced by other bacterial species and therefore plays a significant role in QS [16,17].

Recently, *S. enterica* was used as a carrier to deliver heterologous antigen fusions to stimulate both humoral and cellular immune responses [1,18]. *S. enterica* was engineered to be a candidate for bacteria-mediated tumor therapy [19,20]. The approved safety of *S. enterica* mutants, as well as other factors, makes these bacteria a promising carrier for vaccination against both bacterial, viral infections and cancer, as well [1]. Editing of *S. enterica* chromosome is essential in order to develop new mutant strains which can be used efficiently as carriers for vaccination purposes or used themselves as vaccines [1,19]. Interestingly, affordable and efficient genome editing tools have been developed recently in order to engineer both eukaryotic and prokaryotic organisms.

The CRISPR RNA guided endonuclease is a promising and efficient genome editing tool [21,22]. The CRISPR-Cas system was discovered as a naturally occurring adaptive microbial immune system against invading viruses and other mobile genetic elements [23,24]. Importantly, the CRISPR-Cas9 system was successfully used in targeting the genome of both bacterial [25–28] and eukaryotic cells [29–31]. Mutagenesis introduces a selection marker in the edited locus or requires a process of two steps that includes a counter system for selection [32]. Genome editing tools, such as zinc finger nucleases (ZFN), transcription activator-like effector nucleases (TALENs) and homing meganucleases, have been programmed to cut genomes in specific locations. However, these engineering techniques have been reported to be difficult to use and expensive [25,33].

The CRISPR loci consist of a repeated array of short sequences separated by short spacer sequences; these spacer sequences are complementary to genomes of invading viruses, as well as bacterial and archaeal plasmids [34–37]. The CRISPR-Cas immunity system occurs in three stages: First, Cas proteins integrate short sequences of invading DNA into CRISPR array as a new spacers [38]. Second, as a consequence, the CRISPR array will be transcribed and processed to produce small CRISPR RNAs (crRNAs) that contain a spacer sequence. Finally, crRNAs in association with Cas nucleases target the spacer sequence, leading to its cleavage resulting in destruction of invader's DNA [23,24,39]. There are three major types of prokaryotic CRISPR immune that are grouped according to operon organization and *cas* gene conservation [39]: The type II CRISPR-Cas system is characterized by RNA-guided Cas9 endonuclease activity. It is the simplest of all Cas systems to be used to interfere or even edit both eukaryotic or prokaryotic genomes [31,40,41]. The Cas9 endonuclease activity requires guide sequence (crRNA) to guarantee precise targeting, as well as an immediate downstream motif sequence (PAM). In order to edit the bacterial genome, it is necessary to transfer a vector encoding Cas9 and its guide and recombination template containing the desired mutation [25]. The spacer or PAM sequences must be altered in order to prevent re-cleavage of Cas9 of target genome. This approach has been efficiently used to manipulate several bacterial species [25,26,42].

The current study investigated the effect of *sdiA* mutation on *S. enterica* pathogenesis. The virulence of both *S. enterica* wild type (WT) and Δ*ssaV* mutant is evaluated herein. The *S. enterica* Δ*ssaV* mutant has been studied as a carrier for vaccination [32,43,44]. In addition, *S. enterica* chromosome was edited by using an efficient CRISPR-Cas9 system. Moreover, *sdiA*, which plays an essential role in QS, was targeted in two sites, using Cas9 encoding plasmids in both *S. enterica* WT and *ssaV* mutants. This study aimed to elucidate how much the mutation in *sdiA* and *ssaV* separately, as well as double mutation, would affect *Salmonella* virulence. The influence of *sdiA* mutation on the pathogenesis of both *S. enterica* WT and Δ*ssaV* mutants in early stages of invasion and intracellular survival are characterized. Finally, the effect of *sdiA* mutation on biofilm formation, susceptibility to antibiotics and in vivo pathogenesis are characterized.

2. Materials and Methods

2.1. Bacterial Strains, Plasmids Enzymes, Media and Chemicals

S. enterica serovar Typhimurium NCTC 12023, and the *S.* Typhimurium Δ*ssaV* mutant were kindly provided by Hensel's lab (Germany). Plasmids pCRISPR and pCas9 were obtained from Addgene (http://www.addgene.org/, accessed on 12 May 2021) with No. 42875 and 42876, respectively [25]. Plasmids were introduced into *S. enterica* strains by electroporation, and recombinant strains were cultured in medium containing kanamycin (50 μg/mL), or chloramphenicol (25 μg/mL). All enzymes used to clone CRISPR plasmids and restriction endonuclease were provided from New England Biolabs, USA. Tryptone soy broth (TSB), Tryptic Soy Agar (TSA), Mueller Hinton (MH) broth and agar and Luria–Bertani (LB) broth and agar were purchased from Oxoid (Hampshire, UK). Dulbecco's Modified Eagle's Medium (DMEM) medium was obtained from Sigma-Aldrich (St. Louis, MO, USA). The used N-acylhomoserine lactones is N-hexanoyl-DL-homoserine lactone (CAS Number: 106983-28-2) was ordered from Sigma-Aldrich (St. Louis, MO, USA). All used chemicals were of pharmaceutical grade.

2.2. Targeting sdiA by CRISPR/Cas9

Two plasmids were employed: the first plasmid, pCas9, encodes the Cas9, trcrRNA and crRNA to target guide sequence number 1. The other plasmid, pCRISPR, encodes crRNA for guide sequence number 2 to be targeted by Cas9. It was shown that mutation induction can be facilitated by the co-selection of transformable cells and use of dual-RNA:Cas9 cleavage to induce a small induction of recombination at the target locus. Both plasmids pCas9 and pCRISPR were transformed to competent cells, followed by selection on kanamycin and chloramphenicol-containing LB [25].

The guide sequences shown in Figure 1 were chosen for targeting *sdiA*, using a CRISPER/Cas system. Plasmids pCas9 and pCRISPR were digested by *Bsa*I restriction endonuclease, and digested plasmids were gel-purified. The protocol provided by Addgene was followed to clone a spacer sequence into pCas9 and pCRISPR. Briefly, a spacer sequence of 20 bp was chosen upstream to NGG to be targeted by Cas9 nuclease and was designed with *Bsa*I restriction cut site ends to be ligated directly to *Bsa*I-digested pCas9 and pCRISPR. Oligonucleotides used for plasmids construction are listed in (Table 1). Oligo nucleotides I and II were designed to target the first site, and Oligos III and IV were designed to target the second site (Table 1). The Oligo nucleotides ordered to by synthesized from Sigma Custom DNA Oligos (St. Louis, MO, USA). Oligos I, II, III and IV were phosphorylated using T4 PNK enzyme. Phosphorylated oligo I was annealed to oligo II, and oligo III was annealed to oligo IV in 1M NaCl at 95 °C for 5 min and slowly cooled down to room temperature. Diluted annealed oligos I and II were ligated to *Bsa*I-digested pCas9 plasmid, and the diluted annealed oligos III and IV were ligated to *Bsa*I-digested pCRISPR plasmid. The ligated plasmids to spacer sequences were electroporated sequentially to *S. enterica* WT and Δ*ssaV* mutant competent cells. The transformed cells were grown at 37 °C for 1 h in LB broth containing kanamycin (50 μg/mL) and chloramphenicol (25 μg/mL). Then 100 μL was spread over LB agar containing kanamycin (50 μg/mL) and chloramphenicol (25 μg/mL) and incubated overnight at 37 °C to select the proper clones that harbor the plasmids carrying resistant genes to these antibiotics. For confirmation of proper cloning, the negative colony PCR clones, using oligo I or oligo III, and sdiA-Rev primer were chosen. PCR products were visualized by electrophoresis on agarose gel (0.7%), using 1X TAE (Tris-acetate-EDTA) running buffer at 80–120V, and visualized by 0.5 g/mL ethidium bromide.

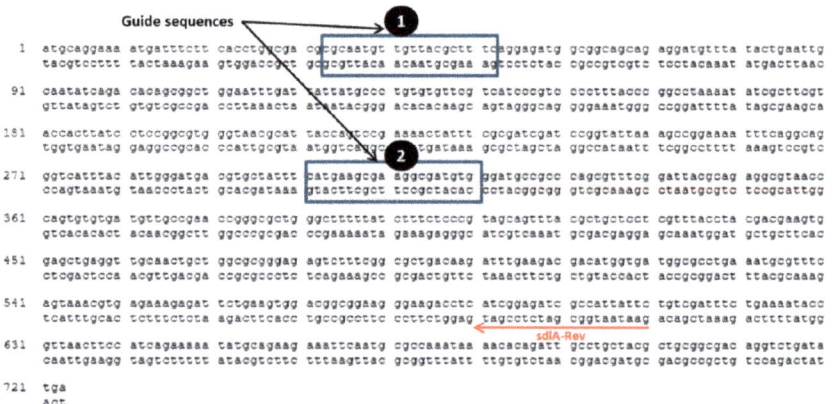

Figure 1. Guide sequences in *S. enterica* serovar Typhimurium NCTC 12023 *sdiA* gene (Gene ID, 1253471; NCBI Reference Sequence, NC_003197.2 (2039655..2040395). Oligo I and II were designed and annealed to target the first guide sequence; oligo III and IV were designed and annealed to target the second sequence site. For confirmation of the mutation in the selected sites, colony PCR was performed by using *sdiA*-Rev and oligo I and III as reverse and forward primers to confirm mutation in first site and second site, respectively.

Table 1. Oligonucleotides used in this study.

Oligonucleotide	Sequence (5′–3′)
Oligo I	AAAC CGCAATGTTGTTACGCTTTC G
Oligo II	AAAAC GAAAGCGTAACAACATTGCG
Oligo III	AAAC CATGAAGCGAAGGCGATGTG G
Oligo IV	AAAAC CACATCGCCTTCGCTTCATG
sdiA-Rev	GAA TAA TGG CGA TCT CCG AT
Seq-primer	CCATAAAATATGCAGGAAA
hSurv-For-EcoRV	TACGATATCGGTGCCCCGACGTTGCCCCC
hSurvivin-HA-Rev-XbaI	ATTTCTAGATTAAGCGTAGTCTGGGACGTCGTAT GGGTAATCCATAGCAGCCAGCTGCTC
SseJ-Pro-For-KpnI	TACGGTACCTCACATAAAACACTAGCAC
SseJ-Rev-EcoRV	ACGGATATCTTCAGTGGAATAATGATGAGC
T7-Seq	TAATACGACTCACTATAGGG
T3-Seq	AATTAACCCTCACTAAAGG

2.3. Adhesion Assay

Overnight cultures of *S. enterica* serovar Typhimurium (*S.* Typhimurium) WT and Δ*ssaV* mutant with or without *sdiA* targeted CRISPR-Cas9 (Δ*sdiA*) strains were prepared, diluted with fresh TSB and adjusted to a cell density of 1×10^6 CFU/mL (OD$_{600}$ = 0.4) for adhesion assay, as previously described [45].

2.3.1. Adhesion to Epithelial Cells

Monolayers of HeLa cells were cultured in 24-well plates in DMEM medium [46,47]. HeLa cells were passaged with 70% confluent and washed with sterile PBS before adhesion assay. Bacterial cultures *S.* Typhimurium WT, Δ*ssaV*, Δ*sdiA* and Δ*ssaV*Δ*sdiA* (1×10^6 CFU/mL) and DMEM with or without N-hexanoyl-DL-homoserine lactone (AHL) in final concentration 0.001 µM were added to wells. Incubation was continued for 1 h at 37 °C. Next, epithelial cells were washed 3 times with PBS and lysed at room temperature for 20 min in Triton X-100 (1%). The bacterial suspensions were serially diluted, plated on TSA and incubated overnight at 37 °C for colony counting. The bacterial counts were used to evaluate adhesion rate. Experiment was performed in triplicate, and the means and standard deviations were calculated.

2.3.2. Adhesion to Abiotic Surface and Biofilm Formation

S. Typhimurium strains; WT, Δ*ssaV*, Δ*sdiA* and Δ*ssaV*Δ*sdiA* were cultured with or without N-hexanoyl-DL-homoserine lactone AHL (0.001 µM) in polystyrene microtiter plate and incubated at 37 °C either for 1 h (for evaluation of adhesion) or for 24 h (for evaluation of biofilm formation) [45,47–49]. Incubated plates were washed gently 3 times with phosphate buffer saline (PBS), fixed at 60 °C for 25 min, stained with crystal violet (0.1%) for 15 min and finally washed with PBS. The adhered crystal violet was extracted with ethanol, and optical densities were measured at 590 nm. The assay was repeated in triplicate, and results were expressed as the means ± standard deviations.

2.4. Invasion Assay and Intracellular Replication

Internalization of *S.* Typhimurium strains within different cell lines was evaluated by using the gentamicin protection assay, as formerly described [50]. Briefly, 24-wells polystyrene plates were seeded with HeLa cells and/or RAW264.7 at cell density of 5×10^5 and 2×10^5 cells/well, respectively. Tested strains WT, Δ*ssaV*, Δ*sdiA* and Δ*ssaV*Δ*sdiA* were subcultured from overnight cultures and incubated at 37 °C for 4 h to induce SPI1 conditions. A master-mix of the inoculum (1×10^5 bacteria/well) multiplicity of infection (MOI 1) for HeLa cell infection or raw macrophage was prepared in DMEM, and 300 µL was added to each well. The bacterial infections were performed in either in the absence or presence of N-hexanoyl-DL-homoserine lactone AHL (0.001 µM). Non-internalized bacteria were washed out with pre-warmed PBS after 30 min, and the adhered extracellular bacteria were killed by incubation in media containing gentamicin (100 µg/mL) for 1 h. For invasion assays, HeLa cells were lysed with 0.1% Triton X-100 for 10 min at 25 °C. To determine intracellular bacteria, the inoculum and the lysates were serially diluted and plated onto Mueller Hinton (MH) plates. The percentage of invading *Salmonella* (1 h against inoculum × 100) was calculated. To assay the intracellular replication, the infected cells were washed with PBS and lysed with TritonX-100 (0.1%) for 10 min in 25 °C at 2 and 16 h post-infection. The inoculum and the lysates were serially diluted and plated onto MH plates. The phagocytosed cells numbers/relative untaken cells (2 h against inoculum × 100) and x-fold intracellular replication (16 h against 2 h) were evaluated.

2.5. The Intracellular Behavior of Salmonella Mutants

2.5.1. Construction of SPI2 Expressing Plasmid

For testing the effectiveness of SPI2-T3SS-dependent translocation, pWSK9 P$_{sseJ}$*sseJ*::hSurvivin::HA plasmid was generated as previously described [18]. The hSurvivin gene was PCR-amplified by employing primers hSurvivin-HA-Rev-*Xba*I and hSurv-For-*Eco*RV, and template plasmid pWSK29 P$_{sseA}$sscBsseF::hSurvivin::HA (provided kindly by Prof. Hensel, University of Osanabrueck, Germany). The obtained hSurvivin and pWSK29 plasmid were digested with *Xba*I and *Eco*RV and ligated together. The *sseJ* gene was PCR-amplified by using SseJ-Rev-*Eco*RV and SseJ-Pro-For-*Kpn*I primers prior to its digestion with *Kpn*I and *Eco*RV. The *sseJ* gene and pWSK29::hSurvivin were digested with *Kpn*I and *Eco*RV and ligated to obtain plasmids pWSK29 P$_{sseJ}$sseJ::hSurvivin::HA. Constructed plasmid was electroporated in *S.* Typhimurium strains WT, Δ*ssaV*, Δ*sdiA* and Δ*ssaV*Δ*sdiA* component cells. Positive clones were selected on LB containing carbenicillin (50 μg/mL). Obtained plasmid was confirmed by colony PCR and diagnostic digestion, and they were sequenced by using T7-Seq and T3-Seq primers [18].

2.5.2. Evaluation of SPI2 Effectors Expression

Plasmid pWsk29 P$_{sseJ}$sseJ::hSurvivin was transferred to WT, Δ*ssaV*, Δ*sdiA* and Δ*ssaV*Δ*sdiA* strains. Tested mutants and expression rates were analyzed as described before [18]. Briefly, tested strains harboring plasmid expressing SPI2 effector protein SseJ-hSurvivin tagged with HA regulated by P*sseJ* promoter were cultured in SPI2-inducing minimal media (PCN-P, pH 5.8). Bacterial cells were collected by centrifugation after 6 h. Equal amounts of bacterial cells were lysed and exposed to SDS-PAGE. Western blots were used to detect HA epitope tag, using fluorescent-labeled secondary antibodies. The signal intensities were measured by using the Odyssey system (Li-Cor) in comparison to control DnaK (cytosolic heat shock protein). The experiment was performed in triplicate, and ratios of HA/DnaK signals were calculated and expressed as means ± standard deviation.

2.5.3. Evaluation of Translocation Efficiency

S. enterica WT, Δ*ssaV*, Δ*sdiA* and Δ*ssaV*Δ*sdiA* provided with constructed plasmid for the expression of HA tagged SPI2 effector were used to infect raw macrophage or HeLa cells in absence or presence of AHL at MOI of 100, as described previously [18]. Briefly, cells were fixed at 16 h after infection; *Salmonella* LPS (rabbit anti-*Salmonella* O1,4,5, Difco, BD) and the HA epitope tag (Roche, Basel, Switzerland) were immuno-stained. The cells were analyzed by microscopy, using a Leica laser-scanning confocal microscope. The fluorescence intensities of tagged protein were detected by J-image program in HeLa cells and macrophages. Infected cells harboring similar number of intracellular bacteria were chosen, and the signal of fluorescence intensities for HA tagged proteins were measured. The mean signal intensities and standard deviations were calculated for at least 30 infected cells per tested strains.

2.6. The Effect on Mutation on Bacterial Susceptibility to Antibiotics

The effect of mutation on susceptibility of tested strains to different antibiotics was characterized by determining both the minimum inhibitory concentrations (MICs) and minimum biofilm inhibitory concentrations (MBICs) of tested antibiotics. These antibiotics include ampicillin, ampicillin/sulbactam, amoxicillin/clavulanic acid, piperacillin, azetronam, imipenem, cephardine, ceftazidime, cefotaxime, cefepime, ciprofloxacin, levofloxacin, gatifloxacin, tobramycin, gentamycin, tetracycline, chloramphenicol and trimethoprim/sulfamethoxazole. The broth microdilution method was employed according to Clinical Laboratory and Standards Institute Guidelines (CLSI, 2015) to determine the MICs of tested strains to different antibiotics [51,52]. MBICs are determined by broth dilution method as described earlier [47,53]. Briefly, the optical densities of overnight cultures from tested strains were adjusted equivalent to 0.5 McFarland standard. Aliquots (100 μL) of the cultures were transferred to the wells of microtiter plates and incubated overnight at 37 °C. The plates were washed with PBS and dried, and serial dilutions of antibiotics in MH broth were added to wells containing adhered biofilms. After overnight incubation at 37 °C, MBICs were considered as the lowest concentrations of antibiotics that showed no visible growth in the wells. Both positive control (inoculated bacteria in broth without addition of antibiotics) and negative control (sterile broth without bacteria) were included in the experiment. The antibiotics susceptibility experiment was repeated in triplicate.

2.7. In Vivo Assessment of the Pathogenesis of Tested Mutants

The influence of *sdiA* mutation on *S. enterica* pathogenesis was characterized in vivo in mice by using the protective assay, as described previously [10,54,55]. Briefly, the cell densities of tested strains overnight cultures were adjusted to approximately 1×10^8 CFU/mL in LB broth. Six groups of female albino mice with similar weights were included in the assay, each containing ten mice. The first and second groups were used as negative controls, where mice were intraperitoneally injected with 100 μL PBS or kept uninoculated. Mice in the third group were injected intraperitoneally with 100 μL of *S.* Typhimurium WT strain. Mice in the fourth, fifth and sixth groups were injected with 100 μL of *S.* Typhimurium Δ*ssaV*, Δ*sdiA* or Δ*ssaV*Δ*sdiA* strains, respectively. Mice in all groups were kept at room temperature, with normal feeding and aeration. Mice survival in each group was recorded daily over 5 successive days and plotted by using the Kaplan–Meier method, and significance (* $p < 0.05$) was calculated by using Log-rank test, GraphPad Prism 5.

2.8. Statistical Analysis

Assays were performed in triplicate, and data are presented as median and range, unless otherwise specified. The differences between *S. enterica* WT and mutant strains were analyzed by a *t*-test, using the GraphPad Prism 5 software. A two-tailed *p*-value < 0.05 was considered statistically significant.

3. Results

3.1. CRISPR/Cas9 System Targets sdiA

S. enterica sdiA was targeted by a CRISPR/Cas9 system. Two guide sequences were chosen carefully to be targeted in order to achieve more efficient interference with *S. enterica sdiA*. Positive clones were selected on LB containing kanamycin and chloramphenicol. In spite of large number of escapers, colony PCR using oligo I or oligo III and sdiA-Rev primers was performed (Figure 2), and negative clones were selected and further tested.

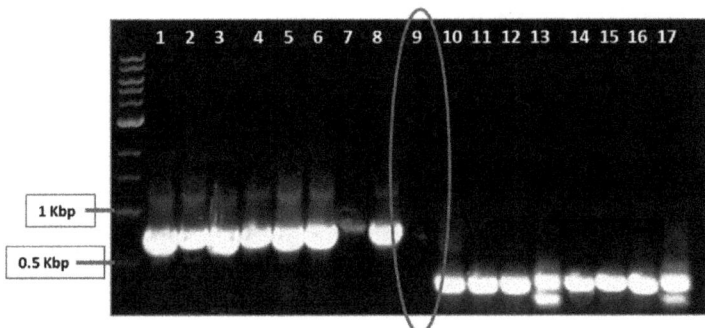

Figure 2. Screening for positive and negative clones, using PCR. Transformed *S. enterica* cells were selected on LB-kanamycin/chloramphenicol plates. Two plasmids were employed herein: The first plasmid, pCas9, encodes the Cas9, trcrRNA and crRNA to target guide sequence number 1. The other plasmid, pCRISPR, encodes crRNA for guide sequence number 2 to be targeted by Cas9. Both plasmids pCas9 and pCRISPR were transformed followed by selection on kanamycin and chloramphenicol-containing LB. However, there were background cells that lack the desired mutation. Colony PCR was performed by targeting both guide sequence 1, using oligo I and *sdiA*-Rev (wells 1–8), and guide sequence 2, using oligo III and *sdiA*-Rev (wells 10–17). Positive PCR clones were omitted, while negative ones (encircled well no. 9) were selected.

3.2. Functional Testing of S. enterica ΔsdiA

It has been shown that *S. enterica* SdiA detects and responds to AHL signals produced by other microbial species [56,57]. The role of SdiA in adhesion [58] and biofilm formation [59] was further characterized. To test the success of targeting *S. enterica sdiA* by CRISPR/Cas9 system, both the adhesion and biofilm-formation capabilities of *Salmonella* Δ*sdiA* were evaluated in comparison with both *S. enterica* WT and Δ*ssaV* strains. Bacterial adhesion to epithelial HeLa cells was performed in both the presence and absence of AHL (Figure 3). *S. enterica* WT, Δ*ssaV* and Δ*sdiA* strains did not exhibit adherence capability to epithelial cells in the absence of AHL. However, the adherence capacity of tested strains significantly increased in the presence of AHL ($p < 0.0001$). In the presence of AHL, the number of adhering *S. enterica* Δ*sdiA* cells was significantly lower than *S. enterica* WT and Δ*ssaV* ($p < 0.0001$). Bacterial adhesion to epithelial cells was not affected by *ssaV* mutation, and the number of adhering cells was not affected in presence of AHL ($p = 0.085$).

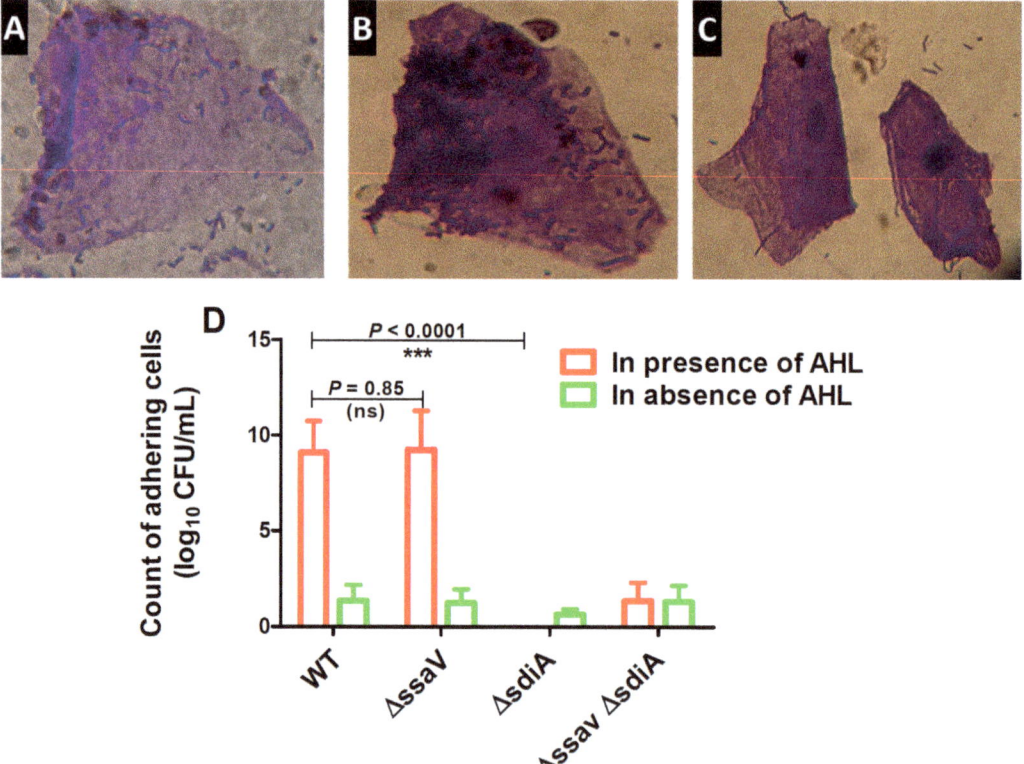

Figure 3. Adhesion of *S. enterica* strains to HeLa cells. HeLa cells were co-cultured with *S. enterica* WT, Δ*ssaV*, Δ*sdiA* or Δ*sdiA* Δ*ssaV* both in the presence and absence of AHL for 1 h at 37 °C. Microscopic examination of crystal violet-stained adhering *S. enterica* to HeLa cells either in presence or absence of AHL. (**A**) *S. enterica* WT adhesion in absence of AHL, (**B**) *Salmonella enterica* WT adhesion in presence of AHL and (**C**) *S. enterica* Δ*sdiA* mutant adhesion in presence of AHL. (**D**) AHL significantly increases adhesion of *S. enterica* WT and Δ*ssaV* but not Δ*sdiA* and Δ*sdiA* Δ*ssaV* mutants to Hela cells. Epithelial cells were lysed with Triton X-100 (1%). Adhering bacteria were serially diluted and counted on agar plates. Experiment was performed in triplicate, and results are represented as means ± standard deviations; *p*-value < 0.05 was considered statistically significant, using a Student's *t*-test (*** = $p < 0.001$).

Moreover, adhesion to abiotic surface and biofilm formation of *S. enterica* WT, Δ*ssaV* and Δ*sdiA* strains were tested both in the presence and absence of AHL (Figure 4). *S. en-*

terica WT, ΔssaV, ΔsdiA and ΔssaVΔsdiA strains were cultured with or without AHL in polystyrene microtiter plate and incubated either for 1 h (for evaluation of adhesion) or for 24 h (for evaluation of biofilm formation). Importantly, AHL significantly increased the adhesion and biofilm formation of both *S. enterica* WT and ΔssaV. Moreover, the adhesion and biofilm formation of *S. enterica* were significantly reduced in *S. enterica* ΔsdiA, as compared with WT and ΔssaV strains both in the presence and absence of AHL ($p < 0.0001$). The current results demonstrate that *S. enterica* adhesion to epithelial cells was not affected by mutation in *ssaV*. Furthermore, bacterial adhesion to abiotic surface and biofilm formation were not influenced by single mutation in *ssaV*.

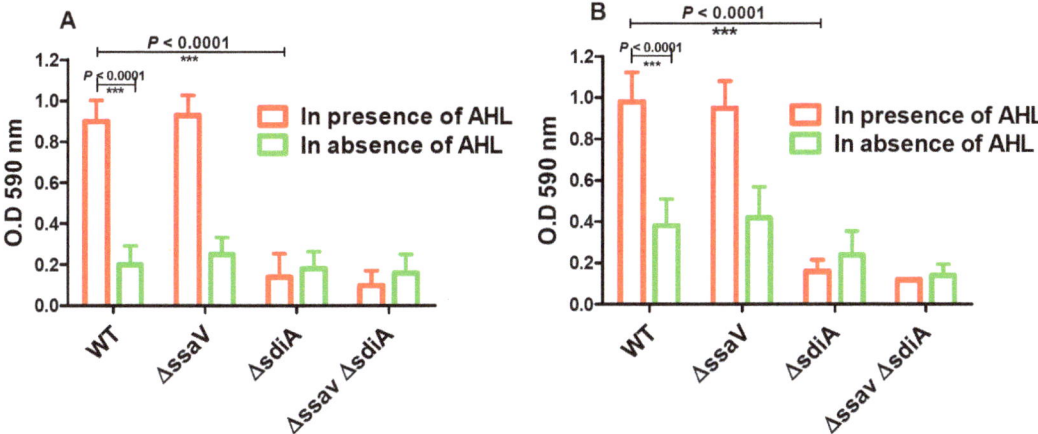

Figure 4. Bacterial adhesion to abiotic surface and biofilm formation. *S. enterica* WT, ΔssaV, ΔsdiA and ΔssaVΔsdiA were cultured in presence or absence of AHL in polystyrene microtiter plate and incubated at 37 °C, either for 1 h (for evaluation of adhesion) or for 24 h (for evaluation of biofilm formation). (**A**) Adhering cells or (**B**) Biofilm forming cells were stained by crystal violet, ethanol was added and optical density was measured at 590 nm. Assays were performed in triplicate, and results were expressed as means ± standard deviations; *p*-value < 0.05 was considered statistically significant, using a two-tailed t-test (*** = $p < 0.001$).

3.3. Intercellular Survival of S. enterica ΔsdiA

S. enterica WT, ΔssaV, ΔsdiA and ΔssaVΔsdiA strains were cultured in SPI1-inducing conditions, and bacterial internalization within HeLa cells or macrophage was assessed by using the gentamicin protection assay. For invasion assays, Hela cells were washed and lysed after 1 h infection with 0.1% Triton X-100 (Figure 5A). The quorum sensing mediator AHL did not increase the invasiveness of *Salmonella* strains. Interference with *sdiA* did not affect bacterial invasiveness either in the absence or presence of AHL. However, AHL did not increase invasiveness of tested strains; the invasiveness of *sdiA* mutant was significantly reduced in comparison to the WT or *ssaV* mutant strain. On the other side, *ssaV* mutation did not influence bacterial invasiveness, as compared to *S. enterica* WT or *sdiA* mutant. For intracellular replication assays, bacteria-infected cells were washed and then lysed with 0.1% Triton-X-100 at 2 and 16 h post-infection (Figure 5B), and intracellular bacteria were counted. Interestingly, AHL did not enhance the invasion of *Salmonella* strains in HeLa cells or bacterial uptake by macrophage. Obviously, *ssaV* mutation significantly decreased the intercellular bacterial replication as compared to the WT and *sdiA* mutant ($p = 0.0062$ and 0.0094; respectively). Moreover, *sdiA* mutation did not increase *Salmonella* intracellular replication within raw macrophage, as compared to *Salmonella* WT ($p = 0.44$).

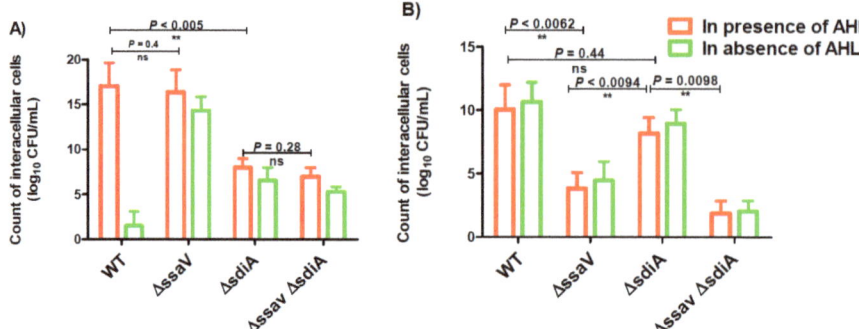

Figure 5. Intercellular survival of *S. enterica* strains in HeLa cells and raw macrophages. *S. enterica* WT, ΔssaV, ΔsdiA and ΔssaVΔsdiA strains were cultured in suitable conditions to induce SPI1 genes. Bacterial strains were used to infect HeLa cells or raw macrophages in multiplicity of infection (MOI of 1). Non-internalized bacteria were removed by washing with PBS, and remaining extracellular bacteria were killed by using gentamicin (100 μg/mL). (**A**) Invasion assays; Hela cells were lysed with 0.1% Triton X-100 after 1 h infection, and intracellular bacteria were counted. The number of invading bacteria (1 h versus inoculum) was calculated. (**B**) Intracellular replication assays; infected cells were lysed with 0.1% Triton-X-100, and intracellular bacteria were counted at 2 and 16 h post-infection. Assays were performed in triplicate, and results were expressed as means ± standard deviations; p-value < 0.05 was considered statistically significant, using a two-tailed t-test (**= p < 0.01).

3.4. Assessment the Expression of SPI2 Effectors S. enterica Strains

To evaluate the capability of tested strains to cope the drastic conditions inside the *Salmonella* containing vacuole (SCV) and survive in order to induce efficient immunologic response, the delivery of SPI2-effector proteins from SCV to outside by live attenuated *Salmonella* mutants (ΔssaV and/or ΔsdiA) was used as indicator. Expression cassettes that contain *sseJ* promoter were constructed with genes encoding SPI2 effector. They were used to express SPI2-T3SS translocated effector proteins SseJ tagged with HA (Figure 6A). In vitro culture conditions were used to induce both the expression of SsrAB regulon and synthesis of SPI2 effector proteins. The synthesis of SPI2-effector fusion protein tagged with HA was quantified (Figure 6B). Western blotting was employed to quantify the amounts of recombinant protein, using the Odyssey detection system and DnaK as control protein. Importantly, the expression level of recombinant protein was significantly reduced in *S. enterica* ΔssaV and ΔsdiA mutants relative to WT.

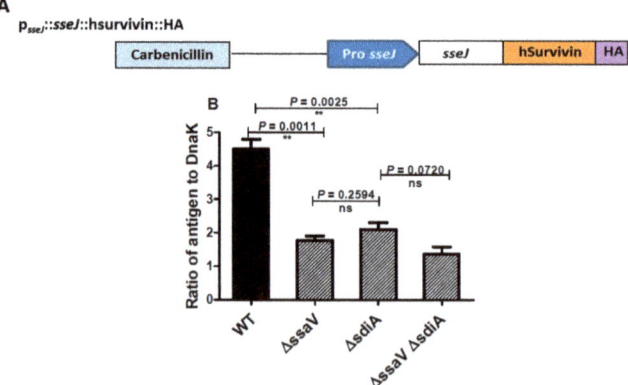

Figure 6. Expression of SPI2 effectors. (**A**) Plasmid-encoding SPI2 effector tagged with HA was constructed in order to test the efficacy of SPI2-TTSS-dependent translocation. (**B**) Expression of translocated proteins was evaluated as ratios of the HA to DnaK signals (**= p < 0.01).

The efficiency of the SPI2-T3SS-dependent translocation in Δ*sdiA* strain was investigated herein. *Salmonella* tested strains harboring the constructed plasmid were used to infect HeLa cells or macrophages (in presence of AHL) and then were processed for immunostaining, and the fluorescence intensities of tagged protein were measured (Figure 7A,B). The translocated proteins were significantly reduced in *S. enterica* Δ*ssaV* and/or sdiA mutants, as compared to WT. Furthermore, the SPI2 effector translocation was significantly reduced in Δ*ssaV* or Δ*ssaV*Δ*sdiA* strains when compared to Δ*sdiA* strains. There was no difference in the SPI2-effector translocation efficacy between *S. enterica* Δ*ssaV* and Δ*ssaV*Δ*sdiA* (Figure 7C,D).

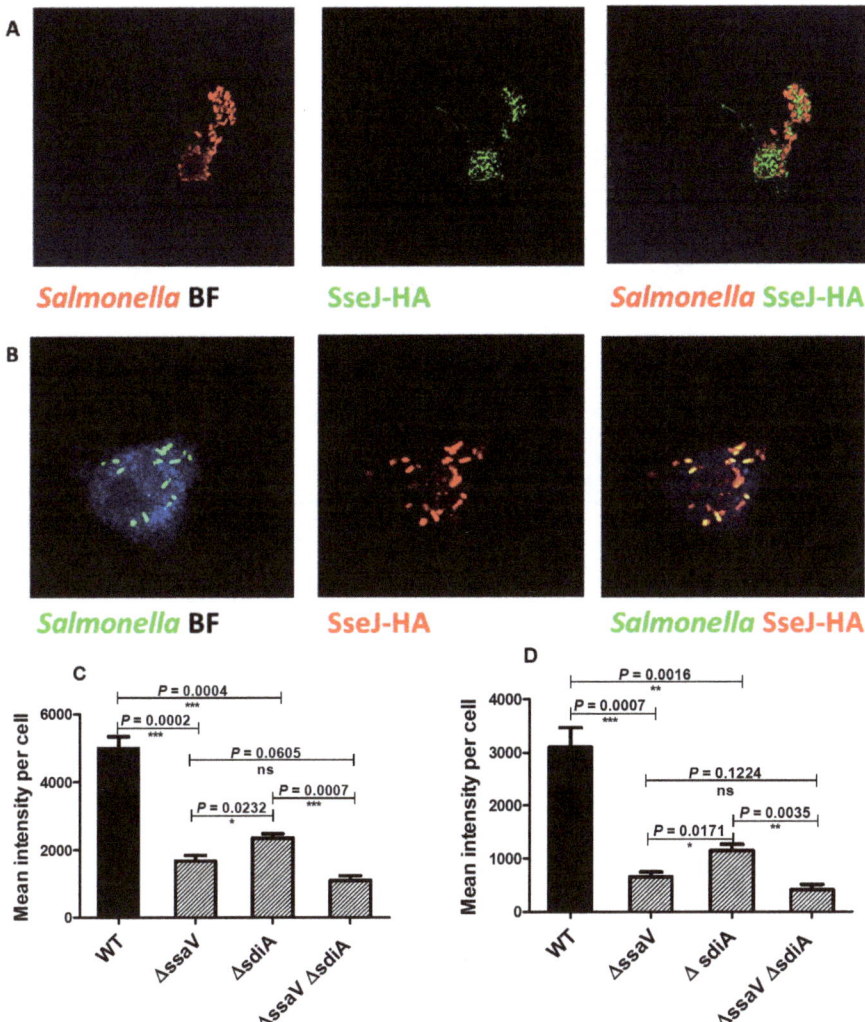

Figure 7. Assessment of SPI2-TTSS translocation of effector proteins. Translocation of SPI2 effectors into the cytoplasm of infected HeLa cells or raw macrophage cells (in presence of AHL) with equal number of *S. enterica* WT, Δ*ssaV*, Δ*sdiA* or Δ*ssaV*Δ*sdiA* harboring constructed plasmid was evaluated. *Salmonella* Lipopolysaccharide (rabbit anti-Salmonella O antigen) and HA epitope tag were immuno-stained and analyzed by Leica laser-scanning confocal microscope both in (**A**) HeLa cells and (**B**) macrophages. Fluorescence intensities of tagged protein were measured by using J-image program both in (**C**) HeLa cells and (**D**) macrophages. (*** = $p < 0.001$; ** = $p < 0.01$; * $p < 0.05$).

3.5. MICs and MBICs of S. enterica Mutant Strains

The influence of the mutations on *S. enterica* resistance to antibiotics was investigated herein. The MICs and MBICs of tested antibiotics were determined by the broth microdilution method, and the results are represented in Table 2. It is shown that the MICs and MBIC were markedly decreased in *S. enterica* ΔssaV, ΔsdiA and ΔssaVΔsdiA mutants in comparison to WT. This indicates that the mutation in *ssaV* and/or *sdiA* genes may increase the susceptibility and decrease the resistance to tested antibiotics.

Table 2. MICs and MBICs (μg/mL) of tested antibiotics against *S.* Typhimurium strains *.

Antibiotic	WT		ΔssaV		ΔsdiA		ΔssaVΔsdiA	
	MIC	MBIC	MIC	MBIC	MIC	MBIC	MIC	MBIC
Ampicillin	256	2048	128	2048	128	1024	64	512
Ampicillin/Sulbactam	128	1024	32	512	32	512	16	128
Amoxicillin/clavulanic acid	128	1024	64	512	32	512	32	256
Piperacillin	32	256	8	32	8	16	8	16
Azetronam	32	512	32	256	16	128	8	128
Imipenem	4	8	2	4	4	4	2	4
Cephardine	64	512	16	256	32	512	16	256
Ceftazidime	32	1024	8	256	8	128	4	64
Cefotaxime	16	256	4	64	4	64	4	64
Cefepime	8	128	4	32	2	16	2	16
Ciprofloxacin	8	12	2	4	2	4	1	2
Levofloxacin	4	16	2	4	1	2	1	2
Gatifloxacin	4	16	2	8	2	8	1	4
Tobramycin	16	512	2	128	2	64	2	64
Gentamycin	16	512	2	64	2	32	2	32
Tetracycline	64	1024	8	512	16	512	8	512
Chloramphenicol	64	1024	16	512	8	256	8	256
Trimehoprim/Sulfamethoxazole	128	2048	64	1024	32	512	16	512

* Statistical analysis by Mann–Whitney U analysis demonstrates a significant difference (* $p < 0.05$) between *S.* Typhimurium WT and mutants (ΔssaV, ΔsdiA and ΔssaVΔsdiA) in their susceptibilities (MICs and MBCs) to tested antibiotics.

3.6. Mutation in sdiA and/or ssaV Genes Decreases S. enterica Virulence In Vivo

The impact of mutation on *S. enterica* virulence was evaluated by using mice infection models. All mice in the negative control groups survived. Similarly, all mice survived in the groups injected with *S. enterica* ΔssaV, ΔsdiA and ΔssaVΔsdiA. On the other side, only five mice out 10 survived in the mice group injected with *S. enterica* WT. The mice survival was observed over five days and plotted by the Kaplan–Meier method, where significance ($p < 0.05$) was assessed by using the Log-rank test (Figure 8). These findings obviously show that the *sdiA* and/or *ssaV* mutations markedly decreased the capacity of *S. enterica* to kill mice ($p = 0.0069$).

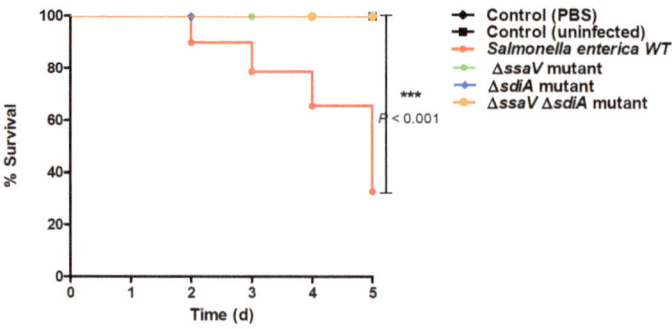

Figure 8. Mutation of *S. enterica sdiA* and/or *ssaV* genes significantly reduced bacterial virulence in mice.

Mice (n = 10 mice/group) were injected with 100 µL of bacterial cells (2×10^6 CFU/mL) of S. Typhimurium WT, ΔssaV, ΔsdiA or ΔssaVΔsdiA strains. No death was reported for mice in negative controls, either uninfected or injected with PBS. Similarly, all mice survived in groups injected with S. enterica ΔssaV, ΔsdiA and ΔssaVΔsdiA. In contrast, mice injected with S. enterica WT showed a higher mortality rate; 5 mice killed out of 10 mice (*** = $p < 0.001$).

4. Discussion

S. enterica is an intracellular bacteria of special interest which could be engineered to deliver heterologous antigens that induce efficient cellular and humoral immune responses [18]. For this purpose, the development of specific mutations in S. enterica chromosome is a critical requirement [1]. In this context, this study aimed to evaluate the influence of sdiA mutation on the virulence of both S. enterica WT and ssaV mutant. The present findings would be valuable and extend our knowledge about employing S. enterica as a vector for delivering antigens and stimulating immune system.

The DNA sequences' altering possibility within the cell in a controlled fashion greatly helps understand gene function. Importantly, the CRISPR prokaryotic immunity system has led to the identification of nucleases whose sequence specificity is programmed by small RNAs [25]. The type II CRISPR-Cas system is characterized by RNA-guided Cas9 endonuclease activity. It is the simplest of all Cas systems to be used to interfere or even edit both eukaryotic and prokaryotic genomes [31,40,41].

In the current work, a CRISPR-Cas9 system approach was used to target S. enterica sdiA, achieving efficient interference with targeted genes in two different sites. The mutation induction can be facilitated by a co-selection of transformable cells and use of dual-RNA:Cas9 cleavage to induce a small induction of recombination at the target locus [25,41]. We tried to edit a Salmonella chromosome to be used as a carrier for vaccination (unpublished data). Lambda red-mediated gene replacement was used to induce specific mutations; however, it was difficult to select proper tetracycline sensitive clones. In comparison, the CRISPR-Cas9 system has the advantage of being more efficient and easier as a bacterial chromosome targeting tool. These results are comparable with those reported in other studies [27,36,37,41,60].

In order to evaluate the role of SdiA in S. enterica pathogenesis at different stages of infection, the sdiA gene was targeted as described in Materials and Methods. S. enterica adhesion to epithelial cells and abiotic surfaces was greatly enhanced in the presence of AHL. Bacterial adhesion is the first step in biofilm formation; as AHL increases bacterial adhesion, the bacterial biofilm formation increases significantly. In order to assess the influence of AHL/SdiA on early stages of S. enterica invasion, the experimental conditions were adjusted to induce SPI1 effectors. As previously mentioned, SdiA is a sensor to AHL; therefore, any mutation or interference within sdiA would impact bacterial QS. S. enterica ΔsdiA lacked the capability to adhere to epithelial cells or abiotic surfaces, and its biofilm formation diminished significantly. The decreased S. enterica biofilm formation upon sdiA mutation relative to WT could account for the lowered MICs and MBICs of tested antibiotics. These findings are in great compliance with several studies that investigated the significant role of SdiA in Salmonella adhesion [15–17,58].

Moreover, S. enterica ΔsdiA exhibited a significant decreased invasion capacity within HeLa cells, regardless the presence or absence of AHL. The present results meet those of an independent work in which the increased bacterial invasion was found to be sdiA-dependent [61]. In addition, SdiA is known to regulate seven genes in S. enterica upon the activation of the SdiA transcription factor by AHL. These genes are located in two different loci: the rck locus and the srgE locus [17]. The rck operon includes srgA, which encodes a disulfide bond oxidoreductase, while SrgA plays a role in folding of fimbrial subunit (PefA) that could affect adhesion [62]. The present findings clearly indicate a role of AHL-SdiA (inducer–receptor) not only in S. enterica adhesion but also in biofilm formation. It is worth mentioning that AHL presence did not enhance S. enterica WT pathogenesis; both bacterial invasion within HeLa cells and intracellular replication in raw macrophage did not increase. However, *S. enterica* invasion was shown to be influenced by *sdiA* mutation, which may lead us to ask if SdiA can be involved directly or indirectly in the SPI1-TTSS functions. Interestingly, current data show that mutation in *sdiA* did not affect *S. enterica* intracellular replication.

Furthermore, the effect of *sdiA* mutation on the functionality of SPI2-TTSS translocation system was explored. The translocation of HA-tagged SPI2-fusion protein in both *S. enterica* WT and Δ*sdiA* mutant was investigated herein. Cells were infected with an equal number of bacteria, and translocated proteins were quantified. Surprisingly, mutation in *sdiA* significantly influenced SPI2 effector translocation. That is in compliance with the fact that *srgA* in *rck* operon, which is regulated by SdiA, plays a role in folding of outer membrane component of SPI2-TTSS [63]. Moreover, the deficient adhesion and invasion may diminish the internalized bacterial cells, and, as a consequence, the expression and translocation may be reduced. SsaV is a vital component for SPI2-TT3SS machinery and essential for secretion of a lot of TTSS effectors [7]. As predicted for *S. enterica* Δ*ssaV*, adherence and invasion within epithelial cells were not affected. In contrast, bacterial intracellular replication and translocation of SPI2 effectors were significantly reduced; these findings are in agreement with previous results [32,43]. For more convenience, the virulence characteristics of *S. enterica* Δ*sdiA*Δ*ssaV* were evaluated. The adhesion, invasion and intercellular replication of the double mutant Δ*sdiA*Δ*ssaV* were greatly diminished, regardless of the presence or absence of AHL. Importantly, double mutation in *sdiA* and *ssaV* genes confers a significate protection to the infected mice.

Attenuated *S. enterica* has been used as a carrier for heterologous antigens, activating both humoral and cellular responses. Previous studies showed that SPI2-T3SS-deficient *S. enterica* was weakened enough and could provide protection from further challenges with WT and induces the production of both secretory IgA and serum IgG against somatic O-antigen in C57BL/6mice [19]. Moreover, *S. enterica* mutants in *ssaV* or any of SPI1-TTSS genes has been efficiently used in preparation of vaccines against typhoid fever [64] or to induce chemokines [65]. On the other hand, *S. enterica* Δ*ssaV* was found to be virulent in immunocompromised C57BL/6 mice [66]. In this study, we showed the ability of tested mutants, especially *S. enterica* Δ*sdiA*Δ*ssaV*, to confer a significant mitigation of *S. enterica* pathogenesis, in comparison with WT or *ssaV* mutant strains. Thus, we need further investigations to evaluate the possibility of using this mutant as a vaccine itself or as a suitable attenuated carrier for heterologous antigens. Targeting bacterial virulence may ease the eradication of virulent bacteria by the host's immune system [5,67].

5. Conclusions

In the current study, a CRISPR-Cas9 system was employed to target bacterial chromosome efficiently. Investigating the virulence characteristics of *S. enterica* Δ*sdiA*Δ*ssaV* demonstrates that *ssaV* mutation did not influence either adherence or invasion of the *S. enterica* Δ*sdiA* strain. Similarly, *sdiA* mutation did not affect the intracellular behavior of Δ*ssaV* strain. These findings could suggest that these two virulence machineries work apart from each other, indicating that *S. enterica* Δ*sdiA*Δ*ssaV* requires more in vivo examination to evaluate its capability to be used as vaccine or carrier for vaccination. SdiA plays a key role in QS as a sensor to signaling AHL. Mutation of *sdiA* significantly affects bacterial adhesion and invasion, as well as biofilm formation. Current data clearly suggest that any agent that reduces SdiA transcription could be used as an antibiofilm agent that could help us control *S. enterica* infection.

Author Contributions: Conceptualization, M.A. and W.A.H.H.; methodology, M.A. and W.A.H.H.; software, A.S.A.L. and E.-S.K.; validation, K.A. and F.A.; formal analysis, A.S.A.L. and E.-S.K.; investigation, T.S.I. and A.J.A. resources, A.S.A.L. and E.-S.K.; data curation, M.A.; T.S.I. and A.J.A. writing—original draft preparation, M.A. and W.A.H.H.; writing—review and editing, M.A. and W.A.H.H.; visualization, M.A. and W.A.H.H.; supervision, W.A.H.H.; project administration, W.A.H.H.; funding acquisition, K.A. and F.A. All authors have read and agreed to the published version of the manuscript.

Funding: This research was funded by the Deanship of Scientific Research (DSR) at King Abdulaziz University, Jeddah, Saudi Arabia under grant no. RG-7-166-42.

Institutional Review Board Statement: This study did not comprise any studies with human participants. The institutional Review Board (ethical committee) at the Faculty of Pharmacy, Zagazig University approved animal experiments in this study. The procedures were performed in compliance with the ARRIVE guidelines, in compliance with the UK Animals (Scientific Procedures) Act, 1986, and related guidelines (ECAHZU, 23 August 2019).

Informed Consent Statement: Not applicable.

Data Availability Statement: Not applicable.

Acknowledgments: The Deanship of Scientific Research (DSR) at King Abdulaziz University, Jeddah, Saudi Arabia funded this project under grant no. RG-7-166-42. The authors, therefore, gratefully acknowledge DSR technical and financial support.

Conflicts of Interest: The authors declare no conflict of interest.

References

1. Hegazy, W.A.H.; Hensel, M. Salmonella enterica as a vaccine carrier. *Futur. Microbiol.* **2012**, *7*, 111–127. [CrossRef]
2. Haraga, A.; Ohlson, M.B.; Miller, S.I. Salmonellae interplay with host cells. *Nat. Rev. Genet.* **2008**, *6*, 53–66. [CrossRef] [PubMed]
3. Ghosh, P. Process of protein transport by the Type III secretion system. *Microbiol. Mol. Biol. Rev.* **2004**, *68*, 771–795. [CrossRef] [PubMed]
4. Gerlach, R.G.; Hensel, M. Salmonella pathogenicity islands in host specificity, host pathogen-interactions and antibiotics resistance of Salmonella enterica. *Berl. Munch. Tierarztl. Wochenschr.* **2007**, *120*, 317–327.
5. Askoura, M.; Hegazy, W.A.H. Ciprofloxacin interferes with Salmonella Typhimurium intracellular survival and host virulence through repression of Salmonella pathogenicity island-2 (SPI-2) genes expression. *Pathog. Dis.* **2020**, *78*, 78. [CrossRef] [PubMed]
6. Deiwick, J.; Salcedo, S.; Boucrot, E.; Gilliland, S.M.; Henry, T.; Petermann, N.; Waterman, S.R.; Gorvel, J.-P.; Holden, D.W.; Méresse, S. The translocated Salmonella effector proteins SseF and SseG interact and are required to establish an intracellular replication niche. *Infect. Immun.* **2006**, *74*, 6965–6972. [CrossRef] [PubMed]
7. Browne, S.H.; Hasegawa, P.; Okamoto, S.; Fierer, J.; Guiney, D.G. Identification of Salmonella SPI-2 secretion system compo-nents required for SpvB-mediated cytotoxicity in macrophages and virulence in mice. *FEMS Immunol. Med. Microbiol.* **2008**, *52*, 194–201. [CrossRef] [PubMed]
8. Wael, A.H.H.; Hisham, A.A.; Hegazy, W.A.H.; Abbas, H.A. Evaluation of the role of SsaV Salmonella pathogenicity island-2 dependent type III secretion system components on the virulence behavior of Salmonella enterica serovar Typhimurium. *Afr. J. Biotechnol.* **2017**, *16*, 718–726. [CrossRef]
9. Abbas, H.A.; Hegazy, W.A.H. Repurposing anti-diabetic drug "Sitagliptin" as a novel virulence attenuating agent in Serratia marcescens. *PLoS ONE* **2020**, *15*, e0231625. [CrossRef] [PubMed]
10. Hegazy, W.A.H.; Khayat, M.T.; Ibrahim, T.S.; Nassar, M.S.; Bakhrebah, M.A.; Abdulaal, W.H.; Alhakamy, N.A.; Bendary, M.M. Repurposing anti-diabetic drugs to cripple Quorum sensing in Pseudomonas aeruginosa. *Microorganisms* **2020**, *8*, 1285. [CrossRef] [PubMed]
11. Askoura, M.; Youns, M.; Hegazy, W.A.H. Investigating the influence of iron on Campylobacter jejuni transcriptome in re-sponse to acid stress. *Microb. Pathog.* **2020**, *138*, 103777. [CrossRef]
12. Li, G.; Yan, C.; Xu, Y.; Feng, Y.; Wu, Q.; Lv, X.; Yang, B.; Wang, X.; Xia, X. Punicalagin inhibits Salmonella virulence factors and has anti-quorum-sensing potential. *Appl. Environ. Microbiol.* **2014**, *80*, 6204–6211. [CrossRef]
13. Jiang, T.; Li, M. Quorum sensing inhibitors: A patent review. *Expert Opin. Ther. Patents* **2013**, *23*, 867–894. [CrossRef]
14. Khayyat, A.; Hegazy, W.; Shaldam, M.; Mosbah, R.; Almalki, A.; Ibrahim, T.; Khayat, M.; Khafagy, E.-S.; Soliman, W.; Abbas, H. Xylitol inhibits growth and blocks virulence in Serratia marcescens. *Microorganism* **2021**, *9*, 1083. [CrossRef] [PubMed]
15. Janssens, J.C.A.; Metzger, K.; Daniels, R.; Ptacek, D.; Verhoeven, T.; Habel, L.W.; Vanderleyden, J.; De Vos, D.E.; De Keersmaecker, S.C.J. Synthesis of N-Acyl Homoserine Lactone analogues reveals strong activators of SdiA, the Salmonella en-terica Serovar Typhimurium LuxR Homologue. *Appl. Environ. Microbiol.* **2007**, *73*, 535–544. [CrossRef] [PubMed]
16. Michael, B.; Smith, J.N.; Swift, S.; Heffron, F.; Ahmer, B.M.M. SdiA of Salmonella enterica is a LuxR Homolog that detects mixed microbial communities. *J. Bacteriol.* **2001**, *183*, 5733–5742. [CrossRef]
17. Smith, J.N.; Ahmer, B.M.M. Detection of other microbial species by Salmonella: Expression of the SdiA regulon. *J. Bacteriol.* **2003**, *185*, 1357–1366. [CrossRef] [PubMed]
18. Hegazy, W.A.H.; Xu, X.; Metelitsa, L.; Hensel, M. Evaluation of Salmonella enterica Type III secretion system effector proteins as carriers for heterologous vaccine antigens. *Infect. Immun.* **2012**, *80*, 1193–1202. [CrossRef] [PubMed]
19. Xu, X.; Hegazy, W.; Guo, L.; Gao, X.; Courtney, A.N.; Kurbanov, S.; Liu, D.; Tian, G.; Manuel, E.; Diamond, D.; et al. Effective cancer vaccine platform based on attenuated Salmonella and a Type III secretion system. *Cancer Res.* **2014**, *74*, 6260–6270. [CrossRef]

20. Theys, J.; Barbe, S.; Landuyt, W.; Nuyts, S.; Mellaert, L.; Wouters, B.; Anné, J.; Lambin, P. Tumor-specific gene delivery using genetically engineered bacteria. *Curr. Gene Ther.* **2003**, *3*, 207–221. [CrossRef] [PubMed]
21. Wiedenheft, B.; Sternberg, S.H.; Doudna, J.A. RNA-guided genetic silencing systems in bacteria and archaea. *Nat. Cell Biol.* **2012**, *482*, 331–338. [CrossRef]
22. Charpentier, E.; Doudna, J.A. Rewriting a genome. *Nat. Cell Biol.* **2013**, *495*, 50–51. [CrossRef]
23. Deveau, H.; Garneau, J.E.; Moineau, S. CRISPR/Cas system and its role in phage-bacteria interactions. *Annu. Rev. Microbiol.* **2010**, *64*, 475–493. [CrossRef] [PubMed]
24. Horvath, P.; Barrangou, R. CRISPR/Cas, the immune system of bacteria and Archaea. *Science* **2010**, *327*, 167–170. [CrossRef] [PubMed]
25. Jiang, W.; Bikard, D.; Cox, D.; Zhang, F.; Marraffini, A.L. RNA-guided editing of bacterial genomes using CRISPR-Cas sys-tems. *Nat. Biotechnol.* **2013**, *31*, 233–239. [CrossRef] [PubMed]
26. Jiang, Y.; Chen, B.; Duan, C.; Sun, B.; Yang, J.; Yang, S. Multigene editing in the Escherichia coli genome via the CRISPR-Cas9 system. *Appl. Environ. Microbiol.* **2015**, *81*, 2506–2514. [CrossRef] [PubMed]
27. Oh, J.-H.; Van Pijkeren, J.-P. CRISPR–Cas9-assisted recombineering in Lactobacillus reuteri. *Nucleic Acids Res.* **2014**, *42*, e131. [CrossRef] [PubMed]
28. Wang, Y.; Zhang, Z.; Seo, S.-O.; Choi, K.; Lu, T.; Jin, Y.-S.; Blaschek, H.P. Markerless chromosomal gene deletion in Clostrid-ium beijerinckii using CRISPR/Cas9 system. *J. Biotechnol.* **2015**, *200*, 1–5. [CrossRef] [PubMed]
29. Lee, J.; Chung, J.-H.; Kim, H.M.; Kim, D.-W.; Kim, H.H. Designed nucleases for targeted genome editing. *Plant. Biotechnol. J.* **2015**, *14*, 448–462. [CrossRef]
30. Xie, K.; Yang, Y. RNA-guided genome editing in plants using a CRISPR–Cas system. *Mol. Plant.* **2013**, *6*, 1975–1983. [CrossRef]
31. Hsu, P.D.; Lander, E.S.; Zhang, F. Development and applications of CRISPR-Cas9 for genome engineering. *Cell* **2014**, *157*, 1262–1278. [CrossRef]
32. Braukmann, M.; Methner, U.; Berndt, A. Immune reaction and survivability of Salmonella Typhimurium and Salmonella Infantis after infection of primary avian macrophages. *PLoS ONE* **2015**, *10*, e0122540. [CrossRef]
33. Hegazy, W.; Youns, M. TALENs construction: Slowly but surely. *Asian Pac. J. Cancer Prev.* **2016**, *17*, 3329–3334.
34. Bolotin, A.; Quinquis, B.; Sorokin, A.; Ehrlich, S.D. Clustered regularly interspaced short palindrome repeats (CRISPRs) have spacers of extrachromosomal origin. *Microbiology* **2005**, *151*, 2551–2561. [CrossRef]
35. Mojica, F.J.M.; Díez-Villaseñor, C.; García-Martínez, J.; Soria, E. Intervening sequences of regularly spaced prokaryotic repeats derive from foreign genetic elements. *J. Mol. Evol.* **2005**, *60*, 174–182. [CrossRef]
36. Pourcel, C.; Salvignol, G.; Vergnaud, G. CRISPR elements in Yersinia pestis acquire new repeats by preferential uptake of bac-teriophage DNA, and provide additional tools for evolutionary studies. *Microbiology* **2005**, *151*, 653–663. [CrossRef] [PubMed]
37. Marraffini, L.A.; Sontheimer, E.J. CRISPR interference limits horizontal gene transfer in Staphylococci by targeting DNA. *Sci-ence* **2008**, *322*, 1843–1845. [CrossRef]
38. Heler, R.; Marraffini, L.A.; Bikard, D. Adapting to new threats: The generation of memory by CRISPR-Cas immune systems. *Mol. Microbiol.* **2014**, *93*, 1–9. [CrossRef]
39. Makarova, K.S.; Haft, D.H.; Barrangou, R.; Brouns, S.J.; Charpentier, E.; Horvath, P.; Moineau, S.; Mojica, F.J.; Wolf, Y.; Ya-kunin, A.; et al. Evolution and classification of the CRISPR–Cas systems. *Nat. Rev. Genet.* **2011**, *9*, 467–477. [CrossRef]
40. Gratz, S.J.; Wildonger, J.; Harrison, M.M.; O'Connor-Giles, K.M. CRISPR/Cas9-mediated genome engineering and the promise of designer flies on demand. *Fly* **2013**, *7*, 249–255. [CrossRef]
41. Jiang, W.; Marraffini, L.A. CRISPR-Cas: New tools for genetic manipulations from bacterial immunity systems. *Annu. Rev. Microbiol.* **2015**, *69*, 209–228. [CrossRef]
42. Huang, H.; Zheng, G.; Jiáng, W.; Hu, H.; Lu, Y. One-step high-efficiency CRISPR/Cas9-mediated genome editing in Strepto-myces. *Acta Biochim. Biophys. Sin.* **2015**, *47*, 231–243. [CrossRef]
43. Fierer, J.; Okamoto, S.; Banerjee, A.; Guiney, D.G. Diarrhea and Colitis in mice require the Salmonella Pathogenicity Island 2-Encoded secretion function but Not SifA or Spv effectors. *Infect. Immun.* **2012**, *80*, 3360–3370. [CrossRef]
44. Li, S.; Zhang, Z.; Pace, L.; Lillehoj, H.; Zhang, S. Functions exerted by the virulence-associated type-three secretion systems during Salmonella enterica serovar Enteritidis invasion into and survival within chicken oviduct epithelial cells and macro-phages. *Avian Pathol.* **2009**, *38*, 97–106. [CrossRef] [PubMed]
45. Vesterlund, S.; Paltta, J.; Karp, M.; Ouwehand, A. Measurement of bacterial adhesion—In vitro evaluation of different meth-ods. *J. Microbiol. Methods* **2005**, *60*, 225–233. [CrossRef]
46. Schmidt, M.; Olejnik-Schmidt, A.K.; Myszka, K.; Borkowska, M.; Grajek, W. Evaluation of quantitative PCR Measurement of bacterial colonization of Epithelial cells. *Pol. J. Microbiol.* **2010**, *59*, 89–93. [CrossRef] [PubMed]
47. Khayyat, A.; Abbas, H.; Mohamed, M.; Asfour, H.; Khayat, M.; Ibrahim, T.; Youns, M.; Khafagy, E.-S.; Abu Lila, A.; Safo, M.; et al. Not only antimicrobial: Metronidazole Mitigates the virulence of Proteus mirabilis isolated from macerated diabetic foot ulcer. *Appl. Sci.* **2021**, *11*, 6847. [CrossRef]
48. Stepanović, S.; Vuković, D.; Dakić, I.; Savić, B.; Švabić-Vlahović, M. A modified microtiter-plate test for quantification of staphylococcal biofilm formation. *J. Microbiol. Methods* **2000**, *40*, 175–179. [CrossRef]
49. Al Saqr, A.; Aldawsari, M.F.; Khafagy, E.-S.; Shaldam, M.A.; Hegazy, W.A.H.; Abbas, H.A. A novel use of Allopurinol as a quorum-sensing inhibitor in Pseudomonas aeruginosa. *Antibiotics* **2021**, *10*, 1385. [CrossRef]

50. Hölzer, S.U.; Hensel, M. Divergent roles of Salmonella Pathogenicity Island 2 and metabolic traits during interaction of S. en-terica Serovar Typhimurium with host cells. *PLoS ONE* **2012**, *7*, e33220. [CrossRef]
51. Aldawsari, M.; Khafagy, E.-S.; Saqr, A.; Alalaiwe, A.; Abbas, H.; Shaldam, M.; Hegazy, W.; Goda, R. Tackling virulence of Pseudomonas aeruginosa by the Natural Furanone Sotolon. *Antibiotics* **2021**, *10*, 871. [CrossRef] [PubMed]
52. Al Saqr, A.; Khafagy, E.-S.; Alalaiwe, A.; Aldawsari, M.; Alshahrani, S.; Anwer, K.; Khan, S.; Lila, A.; Arab, H.; Hegazy, W. Synthesis of gold nanoparticles by using green machinery: Characterization and in vitro toxicity. *Nanomaterials* **2021**, *11*, 808. [CrossRef] [PubMed]
53. Khayyat, A.N.; Abbas, H.A.; Khayat, M.T.; Shaldam, M.A.; Askoura, M.; Asfour, H.Z.; Khafagy, E.-S.; Abu Lila, A.S.; Allam, A.N.; Hegazy, W.A.H. Secnidazole is a promising imidazole mitigator of Serratia marcescens virulence. *Microorganism* **2021**, *9*, 2333. [CrossRef] [PubMed]
54. Hegazy, W.A.; Khayat, M.T.; Ibrahim, T.S.; Youns, M.; Mosbah, R.; Soliman, W.E. Repurposing of antidiabetics as Serratia marcescens virulence inhibitors. *Braz. J. Microbiol.* **2021**, *52*, 627–638. [CrossRef] [PubMed]
55. Bendary, M.M.; Ibrahim, D.; Mosbah, R.A.; Mosallam, F.; Hegazy, W.A.H.; Awad, N.F.S.; Alshareef, W.A.; Al Omar, S.Y.; Zaitone, S.A.; El-Hamid, M.I.A. Thymol Nanoemulsion: A new therapeutic option for extensively drug resistant foodborne pathogens. *Antibiotics* **2020**, *10*, 25. [CrossRef]
56. Rychlik, I.; Barrow, P.A. Salmonella stress management and its relevance to behaviour during intestinal colonisation and infec-tion. *FEMS Microbiol. Rev.* **2005**, *29*, 1021–1040. [CrossRef] [PubMed]
57. Soares, A.J.; Ahmer, B.M. Detection of acyl-homoserine lactones by Escherichia and Salmonella. *Curr. Opin. Microbiol.* **2011**, *14*, 188–193. [CrossRef]
58. Smith, J.N.; Dyszel, J.L.; Soares, J.A.; Ellermeier, C.D.; Altier, C.; Lawhon, S.D.; Adams, L.G.; Konjufca, V.; Curtiss, R.; Slauch, J.M.; et al. SdiA, an N-Acylhomoserine lactone receptor, becomes active during the transit of Salmonella enterica through the gastrointestinal tract of turtles. *PLoS ONE* **2008**, *3*, e2826. [CrossRef] [PubMed]
59. Liu, Z.; Que, F.; Liao, L.; Zhou, M.; You, L.; Zhao, Q.; Li, Y.; Niu, H.; Wu, S.; Huang, R. Study on the promotion of bacterial biofilm formation by a Salmonella Conjugative Plasmid and the Underlying mechanism. *PLoS ONE* **2014**, *9*, e109808. [CrossRef]
60. Marraffini, L.A.; Sontheimer, E.J. CRISPR interference: RNA-directed adaptive immunity in bacteria and archaea. *Nat. Rev. Genet.* **2010**, *11*, 181–190. [CrossRef]
61. Nesse, L.L.; Berg, K.; Vestby, L.K.; Olsaker, I.; Djønne, B. Salmonella Typhimurium invasion of HEp-2 epithelial cells in vitro is increased by N-acylhomoserine lactone quorum sensing signals. *Acta Vet. Scand.* **2011**, *53*, 44. [CrossRef] [PubMed]
62. Bouwman, C.W.; Kohli, M.; Killoran, A.; Touchie, G.A.; Kadner, R.J.; Martin, N.L. Characterization of SrgA, a Salmonella en-terica Serovar Typhimurium virulence plasmid-encoded paralogue of the Disulfide Oxidoreductase DsbA, essential for bio-genesis of plasmid-encoded fimbriae. *J. Bacteriol.* **2003**, *185*, 991–1000. [CrossRef] [PubMed]
63. Miki, T.; Okada, N.; Danbara, H. Two periplasmic disulfide oxidoreductases, DsbA and SrgA, target outer membrane protein SpiA, a component of the Salmonella Pathogenicity Island 2 Type III secretion system. *J. Biol. Chem.* **2004**, *279*, 34631–34642. [CrossRef] [PubMed]
64. Pati, N.B.; Vishwakarma, V.; Selvaraj, S.K.; Dash, S.; Saha, B.; Singh, N.; Suar, M. Salmonella Typhimurium TTSS-2 deficient mig-14 mutant shows attenuation in immunocompromised mice and offers protection against wild-type Salmonella Typhi-murium infection. *BMC Microbiol.* **2013**, *13*, 236. [CrossRef] [PubMed]
65. Li, S.; Zhang, M.Z.; Yan, L.; Lillehoj, H.; Pace, L.W.; Zhang, S. Induction of CXC Chemokine messenger-RNA expression in chicken oviduct epithelial cells by Salmonella enterica serovar Enteritidis via the type three secretion system–1. *Avian Dis.* **2009**, *53*, 396–404. [CrossRef]
66. Periaswamy, B.; Maier, L.; Vishwakarma, V.; Slack, E.; Kremer, M.; Andrews-Polymenis, H.L.; McClelland, M.; Grant, A.J.; Suar, M.; Hardt, W.-D. Live attenuated S. Typhimurium vaccine with improved safety in immuno-compromised mice. *PLoS ONE* **2012**, *7*, e45433. [CrossRef]
67. Aldawsari, M.; Alalaiwe, A.; Khafagy, E.-S.; Al Saqr, A.; Alshahrani, S.; Alsulays, B.; Alshehri, S.; Abu Lila, A.; Rizvi, S.D.; Hegazy, W. Efficacy of SPG-ODN 1826 Nanovehicles in inducing M1 phenotype through TLR-9 activation in murine alveolar J774A.1 cells: Plausible nano-immunotherapy for lung carcinoma. *Int. J. Mol. Sci.* **2021**, *22*, 6833. [CrossRef] [PubMed]

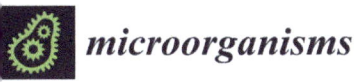

Article

Bacterial Morphotypes as Important Trait for Uropathogenic *E. coli* Diagnostic; a Virulence-Phenotype-Phylogeny Study

Manuel G. Ballesteros-Monrreal [1], Margarita M. P. Arenas-Hernández [2], Edwin Barrios-Villa [3], Josue Juarez [4], Maritza Lizeth Álvarez-Ainza [1], Pablo Taboada [5], Rafael De la Rosa-López [3], Enrique Bolado-Martínez [1,*] and Dora Valencia [3,*]

[1] Departamento de Ciencias Químico-Biológicas, Universidad de Sonora, Hermosillo C.P. 83000, Sonora, Mexico; manuel.ballesteros@unison.mx (M.G.B.-M.); maritza.alvarez@unison.mx (M.L.Á.-A.)

[2] Posgrado en Microbiología, Centro de Investigación en Ciencias Microbiológicas, Instituto de Ciencias, Benemérita Universidad Autónoma de Puebla, Ciudad Universitaria, Puebla C.P. 72590, Pue, Mexico; margarita.arenas@correo.buap.mx

[3] Departamento de Ciencias Químico-Biológicas y Agropecuarias, Universidad de Sonora, Caborca C.P. 83621, Sonora, Mexico; edwin.barrios@unison.mx (E.B.-V.); rafael.delarosa@unison.mx (R.D.l.R.-L.)

[4] Departamento de Física, Universidad de Sonora, Hermosillo C.P. 83000, Sonora, Mexico; josue.juarez@unison.mx

[5] Grupo de Física de Coloides y Polímeros Departamento de Física de Partículas, Universidad de Santiago de Compostela, C.P. 15782 Santiago de Compostela, Spain; pablo.taboada@usc.es

* Correspondence: enrique.bolado@unison.mx (E.B.-M.); dora.valencia@unison.mx (D.V.); Tel.: +52-(662)-259-21-63 (E.B.-M.); +52-(637)-372-65-40 (D.V.)

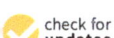

Citation: Ballesteros-Monrreal, M.G.; Arenas-Hernández, M.M.P.; Barrios-Villa, E.; Juarez, J.; Álvarez-Ainza, M.L.; Taboada, P.; De la Rosa-López, R.; Bolado-Martínez, E.; Valencia, D. Bacterial Morphotypes as Important Trait for Uropathogenic *E. coli* Diagnostic; a Virulence-Phenotype-Phylogeny Study. *Microorganisms* **2021**, *9*, 2381. https://doi.org/10.3390/microorganisms9112381

Academic Editor: Dobroslava Bujňáková

Received: 26 October 2021
Accepted: 13 November 2021
Published: 18 November 2021

Publisher's Note: MDPI stays neutral with regard to jurisdictional claims in published maps and institutional affiliations.

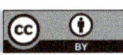

Copyright: © 2021 by the authors. Licensee MDPI, Basel, Switzerland. This article is an open access article distributed under the terms and conditions of the Creative Commons Attribution (CC BY) license (https://creativecommons.org/licenses/by/4.0/).

Abstract: Urinary tract infections (UTIs) belong to the most common pathologies in Mexico and are mainly caused by Uropathogenic *Escherichia coli* (UPEC). UPEC possesses a wide diversity of virulence factors that allow it to carry out its pathogenesis mechanism in the urinary tract (UT). The development of morphotypes in UT represents an important feature of UPEC because it is associated with complications in diagnosis of UTI. The aim of this study was to determine the presence of bacterial morphotypes, virulence genes, virulence phenotypes, antibiotic resistant, and phylogenetic groups in clinical isolates of UPEC obtained from women in Sonora, Mexico. Forty UPEC isolates were obtained, and urine morphotypes were observed in 65% of the urine samples from where *E. coli* was isolated. Phylogenetic group B2 was the most prevalent. The most frequent virulence genes were *fimH* (100%), *fliCD* (90%), and *sfaD/focC* (72%). Biofilm formation (100%) and motility (98%) were the most prevalent phenotypes. Clinical isolates showed high resistance to aminoglycosides and β-lactams antibiotics. These data suggest that the search for morphotypes in urine sediment must be incorporated in the urinalysis procedure and also that clinical isolates of UPEC in this study can cause upper, lower, and recurrent UTI.

Keywords: urinary tract infection; UPEC morphotypes; UPEC virulence

1. Introduction

Urinary tract infections (UTIs) are one of the most common pathologies in Mexico with more than 4 million cases reported each year [1,2]. Although UTIs are common in both males and females, the prevalence is higher in women (>70%). In this regard, it is estimated that 50% of all women worldwide will present at least one episode of UTI in their lives, and 30% of this population will experience recurrent episodes [3,4].

The etiology of UTI is varied; however, the main causative pathogen of this condition is uropathogenic *Escherichia coli* (UPEC) [3,4]. In contrast to other *E. coli* pathotypes, UPEC does not possess a specific virulence profile, but its virulence genes are mainly associated with characteristics such as adherence, motility, iron capture, and toxigenicity. These virulence features allow UPEC to adapt and carry out successfully its pathogenesis mechanism in the urinary tract [5–7]. In this sense, one of the most important virulence traits of UPEC is its adherence capacity: it is known that the fimbrial adhesin FimH allows the pathogen not only to adhere to the bladder, but also favors its internalization in the target cell forming biofilm-like communities, denominated intracellular bacterial communities (IBC), which are associated with persistence in the urinary tract, antimicrobial resistance, and recurrent UTI [4,8]. In addition to IBC, UPEC can also form biofilm and filamentous bacteria in the urinary tract, which are implicated in antimicrobial resistance and immune evasion. In the clinical environment, the presence of these, also called bacterial morphotypes, in urinary sediments is important since they could be used as an additional valuable tool in the microbiological diagnosis of UTI due to UPEC [4,9–11].

On the other hand, it is known that *Escherichia coli* can be phylogenetically classified into seven phylogenetic groups (A, B1, B2, C, D, E, and F). Among these groups, B2 and D are those associated with pathogenic strains for humans, while groups A and B1 are related to both commensal and antibiotic resistance strains [12,13]. However, a high prevalence of UPEC belonging to phylogenetic groups considered to be non-pathogenic has been observed causing disease, which besides their multidrug resistance, also show a significant number of virulence associated genes [14–16].

Urinary tract infections represent the third most common cause of morbidity in Mexico. Despite its importance, there is little evidence focused on UPEC and its virulence characteristics. The knowledge of the prevalent virulence features in clinical isolates of UPEC will allow us to better understand its pathogenesis mechanisms and its possible implication in the improvement of the diagnosis and treatment of UTI. In this context, the aim of this work is to determine the more prevalent phylogenetic groups, virulence genes, virulence phenotypes, antibiotic resistant, and bacterial morphotypes of clinical isolates of UPEC recovered from women in Mexico.

2. Materials and Methods

2.1. Urine Samples Collection

Urine samples were collected from outpatients assisted in a public hospital in Sonora, Mexico, following aseptic directions. Male patients, children, and those who refused to give consent were not included in the study. Clinical data (age, signs, and symptoms, UTI recurrence, antibiotics treatments, and functional or morphological abnormalities in urinary tract) were collected in a survey. Patient data were maintained under anonymity.

2.2. Urinalysis and Detection of UPEC Morphotypes in Urine Sediment

The obtained urine samples were examined using URISPIN-U120 (Spinreact, Girona, Spain) with URIN-10 (Spinreact, Girona, Spain) dipsticks. For UPEC morphotypes detection, 10 mL of urine were centrifuged for 10 min at $400 \times g$. The urine sediment was examined microscopically using Sternheimmer-Malbin stain. Samples were considered as positive for presence of morphotype if adherence, IBC, or filamentous bacteria were observed. According to previously proposed criteria and morphologic characteristics, adherence phenotype was considered positive when bacteria attached to epithelial cells were observed, while detection of dark-pink staining cells with suggestive images of intracellular bacteria and filamentous bacteria was considered as positive for IBC and *E. coli* filamentation, respectively [11,17].

2.3. Urine Cultures and Biochemical Identification of Obtained Bacterial Isolates

Urine samples were inoculated (1 µL with a sterile loop) on MacConkey agar and Mannitol-Salt agar for microbiological analysis. For CFU/mL count, samples were seeded on Trypticase Soy Agar (TSA) using a calibrated loop (0.001 mL). If morphotypes were observed, 10 mL of urine sample were vortexed for 1 min to release intracellular bacteria and seeded on additional TSA plate for CFU counts. Cultures were incubated for 18–24 h at 37 °C.

Uropathogens were identified by IMViC tests (indole, methyl red, vogues-Proskauer, and citrate production). In addition, urease, lysine decarboxylase, and ornithine decarboxylase production were included. Clinical isolates that were not identified as *E. coli* were reported but were not considered in this study.

If the patients had symptoms of UTI or bacterial morphotypes were observed in urine sediment, less than 10^5 CFU/mL were considered as positive for urine culture [18].

2.4. DNA Extraction

Bacterial DNA was obtained by alkaline lysis, according to protocols previously reported [19].

2.5. Molecular Identification of E. coli

Clinical isolates were confirmed by polymerase chain reaction (PCR) using primers for the *ybbW* gene that encodes for an allantoin receptor, which is highly specific for *E. coli* [20]. The PCR product was observed by electrophoresis on a 2% agarose gel in 1× TAE buffer stained with GelStarTM Stain (Lonza, Morristown, NJ, USA).

2.6. Identification of Phylogenetic Groups

The method described by Clermont et al. 2013 was used to identify the phylogenetic group. This method is based on detection of *arpA*, *chuA*, *yjaA*, and *TspE4.C2* genes by using a quadruplex PCR [13].

2.7. Genotypic Characterization of UPEC Isolates

Virulence associated genes were identified by multiplex polymerase chain reaction (mPCR). Eighteen genes were investigated in six multiplex PCR: mPCR 1 (Adherence associated genes): *fimH* (type 1 pilus adhesin), *sfaD/focC* (S and Dra fimbriae), *papG-II* (type P pilus adhesin allele 2), and *papC* (type P pilus chaperone); mPCR 2 (Motility and toxigenicity associated genes): *fliCD* (flagella), *sat* (autotransporter secreted toxin); mPCR 3 (Immune evasion and toxigenicity associated genes): *kpsM* (capsule) and *hlyA* (α-hemolysin); mPCR 4 (immune evasion and toxigenicity associated genes): *traT* (serum resistance protein), *agn43* (43 antigen), *vat* (vacuolating autotransporter toxing), *cnf-1* (necrotizing cytotoxic factor); mPCR 5 (iron uptake associated genes): *fyuA* (ferric yersiniabactin uptake receptor), *iucD* (aerobactin), *iroN* (salmocheline receptor); mPCR 6 (iron uptake associated genes): *iutA* (aerobactin receptor), *feoB* (ferrous iron transporter), *iha* (irgA homologue Adhesin/enterobactin receptor). *E. coli* CFT073, *E. coli* ATCC 25922, and *E. coli* GAGI were used as a positive control for all evaluated genes. Control strains *E. coli* CFT073 and *E. coli* GAGI were kindly donated by Ph.D. Margarita MP Arenas-Hernández from Centro de Investigación en Ciencias Microbiológicas, Instituto de Ciencias, Benemérita Universidad Autónoma de Puebla. Primer sequences, length of their amplified products, and annealing temperature (Tm °C) are listed in Table 1.

Each PCR reaction was performed using a master mix containing 2 µL of buffer solution, 0.5 µL of a dNTP mixture (10 mM each one), 1.5 µL of 25 mM MgCl$_2$, 0.5 µL of each primer (10 µM), 0.1 µL of GoTaq® Flexi DNA Polymerase (Promega), 1.5 µL [50–75 ng] of template DNA, and necessary distilled water to obtain a final volume of 15.5 µL. Reactions were performed in ProFlex™ PCR System (Thermo Fisher, Waltham, MA, USA). Conditions implemented were: One cycle at 95 °C for 4 min, 35 cycles at 95 °C for 1 min and 10 s, 72 °C for 1 min, and 1 cycle at 72 °C for 10 min. Annealing temperature (Tm °C) and times of reactions were 54 °C for 1 min and 10 s (mPCR 1), 60 °C for 1 min (mPCR 2), 58 °C for 1 min (mPCR 3 and mPCR 4), and 60 °C for 45 s (mPCR 5 and mPCR 6). PCR products were observed by electrophoresis on a 2% agarose gel in 1× TAE buffer stained with GelStarTM Stain (Lonza, USA).

Table 1. Primers used for the detection of virulence associated genes and molecular identification of clinical isolates of *E. coli*.

Gene	Sequence (5′-3′)	Size Product	Tm °C	Reference
fimH	Forward: TTATGGCGGCGTGTTATC Reverse: TCCCTACTGCTCCTAACG	545 bp	54	This study
sfaD/focC	Forward: AGGCAAATGGACAGGTATGG Reverse: TCACCCAGAACAAACTTTCC	412 bp		This study
papG-II	Forward: ATTCACCATAGAGGCGACTG Reverse: ATCATTATGCGGCTCAGAC	237 bp		This study
papC	Forward: TTCTCTCTCCCTCAATACGG Reverse: TTATAACCTCAACGGGACGG	926 bp		This study
fliCD	Forward: CCGAATCAGAGTTAGTTCCG Reverse: CCCAGCGATGAAATACTTGC	610 bp	60	This study
sat	Forward: GTTGGCAAACAGGTCAAAC Reverse: CTCGGAGTATTGGCTTCAG	809 bp		This study
hlyA	Forward: GATACGCTGATAGGTGAG Reverse: CCAGGTGTGACTCAATAC	564 bp	58	This study
kpsM	Forward: CCAGAGTAGATATGACCAG Reverse: CTACGAGAAATACGAACAC	409 bp		This study
agn43	Forward: CACACAGCCACTAATACC Reverse: CACCTGAATACCCTTACC	488 bp		This study
vat	Forward: ATACAGTCTCGTCTCTGG Reverse GTGACAGTCCCTTTATCC	670 bp	58	This study
cnf-1	Forward: CAGACTCATCTTCACTCG Reverse: AGACAGAGACCTTACGAC	551 bp		This study
traT	Forward: TGGTATAGTTCACATCTTCC Reverse: TAAAGCCTACTACTGGATTC	233 bp		This study
fyuA	Forward: CGCCAGTAAACAATCTTCCC Reverse: CCCAAACACCATATCAACGG	937 bp		This study
iucD	Forward: CGTGAGACCCAGTTTATTTCC Reverse: GGGCTGCTGAAGATATGAATAACC	334 bp		This study
iroN	Forward: CAGAATGATGCGGTAACTCC Reverse: CGTGAGACCCAGTTTATTTCC	435 bp		This study
iutA	Forward: GTTCACGCTCTTTGTCAGG Reverse: GGGCTTAATCTCGGGAAAGG	801 bp	60	This study
feoB	Forward: GTCTAACCTTGAGCGTAACC Reverse: GGCGAGGAAGATAGTCAGC	736 bp		This study
iha	Forward: TGTGCTCTGGTTTGATATGG Reverse: CATTCTGGGTGCCTTATATCC	594 bp		This study
ybbW	Forward: TGATTGGCAAAATCTGGCCG Reverse: ATACTGGCAATCAGTACGCC	667 bp		[20]

fimH: Type 1 pilus Adhesin; *sfaD/focC*: S and Dra fimbriae; *papC*: Type P pilus chaperone; *papG-II*: Type P pilus Adhesin allele 2; *fliCD*: Flagellin subunit/flagellar cap; *hlyA*: α-hemolysin; *kpsM*: Capsular variant; *sat*: Autotransporter secreted toxin; *agn43*: Antigen 43; *vat*: Vacuolating autotransporter toxin; *cnf-1*: Necrotizing cytotoxic factor; *traT*: Complement resistance associated protein; *fyuA*: Ferric yersiniabactin uptake receptor; *iucD*: Aerobactin; *iroN*: Salmocheline receptor; *iutA*: Aerobactin receptor; *feoB*: Ferrous iron transporter; *iha*: IrgA homologue Adhesin/enterobactin receptor; *ybbW*: Allantoin receptor.

2.8. Phenotypic Characterization of UPEC Isolates

2.8.1. Motility Test

A 24 h pre-culture of the bacterial isolate was obtained on nutrient agar. For motility detection, tubes with semisolid agar (SIM) were used, UPEC isolates were inoculated with a single stab of an inoculating loop and incubated for 18–24 h at 37 °C. A positive phenotype showed growth away from the stab line of inoculation, evidenced by turbidity. While a negative result is defined by confined growth in the stab line. *E. coli* CFT073 (positive phenotype) and *E. coli* EDL 933 (negative phenotype) were used as a control in each experiment.

2.8.2. α-Hemolysin Production

Twenty-five microliters of a 24 h pre-culture in Luria-Bertani broth (LB) of each UPEC isolate were inoculated in a previously created well in 5% sheep blood agar plate and incubated for 24 h at 37 °C. The presence of hemolysis around the inoculated well was considered as a positive phenotype. *Escherichia coli* CFT073 was used as a positive control, while culture media without bacteria was used as a negative control [14].

2.8.3. Biofilm Formation Assay

The ability to produce biofilm was determined following established protocols with slight modifications [21]. A 24 h preculture of UPEC in Mueller-Hinton Broth supplemented with 1% of glucose was diluted 1:100. Five hundred µL of this dilution were deposited in a microtube and incubated for 24 h at 37 °C. After incubation, planktonic bacteria were removed by gently aspired using a micropipette, washed twice with phosphate buffer saline pH 7.2 (PBS), and fixed with 500 µL of sodium acetate (2% w/v) for 20 min. After that, the microtube was washed again with PBS and stained with 500 µL of crystal violet (0.5% w/v) for 15 min. The remaining crystal violet was removed, and the microtube was washed with water until clearance. Finally, 500 µL of acetic acid (30% v/v) were used to resuspend the crystal violet, and 100 µL were deposited in a polystyrene 96 well plate for optical density reading at 550 nm with an ELISA plate reader (Multiskan EX, ThermoLabSystem, Waltham, MA, USA). *E. coli* ATCC 25,922 was used as a control. Previously established criteria were used to grade the isolates in different biofilm-producing groups based on the optical density (OD) obtained: OD (problem isolate) ≤ ODc (control strain) = no biofilm producer, ODc < OD ≤ 2x ODc = moderate biofilm producer, 4x ODc < OD = strong biofilm producer [22]

2.8.4. Capsule Production

The capsule phenotype was identified using Anthony's stain method. One bacterial colony of each isolate from a 48 h pre-culture on LB agar was deposited onto a glass slide, one drop of physiological solution was added, mixed, and dried at room temperature. The sample was stained with 1% of crystal violet for 1 min and washed with a 20% (w/v) copper sulphate solution and observed by light field microscopy. The presence of a faint blue halo around a purple cell was indicative of positive capsule phenotype. *Escherichia coli* CFT073 was used as a positive control [23].

2.8.5. Adherence Assay

Twenty clinical isolates with the higher number of adherence associated genes (*fimH*, *fliCD*, *sfaD/focC*, *papG-II*, *kpsM*, *iha*, *papC*, and *agn43*) (Supplementary Material Table S1), with biofilm- or capsule-producing phenotypes, and morphotypes in urinary sediment were randomly selected. Additionally, 3–5 clinical isolates from each phylogenetic group were included. HeLa cells were seeded on culture plates in Dulbecco's Modified Eagle Medium (DMEM) (SIGMA) supplemented with 5% fetal bovine serum (FBS) (GIBCO) and incubated at 37 °C in 5% CO_2 until sub-confluence. Six-well polystyrene plates with coverslips were used, and a cellular suspension of 5×10^4 cells/mL was prepared in 2 mL DMEM supplemented with 10% FBS without antibiotics. Plates were then incubated overnight at 37 °C in 5% CO_2. HeLa cells monolayers were washed with sterile PBS. After washing, 2 mL of fresh DMEM supplemented with 10% FBS were added to each well. From an 18–24 h pre-culture in Brain Heart Infusion Broth (BHI) of the problem bacterial isolate, an adjustment was made to 0.5 on the McFarland scale in DMEM and 15 µL of this suspension was placed in contact with the HeLa cells (30:1, Bacteria: HeLa). The plate was then incubated at 37 °C and 5% CO_2 for 3 h. Then, the cells were washed with PBS to remove unattached bacteria, fixed with methanol, stained with Giemsa, washed with PBS three times, and finally, coverslips were removed and mounted on a slide for microscopic observation. *Escherichia coli* strain EDL 933 (EHEC) was used as a positive control. Each clinical isolate was evaluated in three independent experiments by triplicate.

Total HeLa cells and adherent bacteria were counted in 10 fields at 40X objective. The results are expressed as the average number of adherent bacteria. Isolates were classified as low adherent- ($\leq$3 bacteria/HeLa cell), moderately adherent- (4–7 bacteria/HeLa cell), and highly adherent- ($\geq$8 bacteria/HeLa cell) [24,25].

2.8.6. Antibiotic Resistance

Twenty-one antibiotics from twelve categories were tested by disk diffusion method following directions stablished in the Clinical and Laboratory Standards Institute (CLSI, 2021). Antibiotic tested in this study were: Aminoglycosides: Amikacin (AMK, 30 µg), Gentamicin (GM, 10 µg); Fluoroquinolones: Ciprofloxacin (CIP, 5 µg), Levofloxacin (LVX, 5 µg), Norfloxacin (NOR, 10 µg); Sulphas: Cotrimoxazole (TSX, 1.25/23.75 µg); Nitrofurans: Nitrofurantoin (MAC, 300 µg); Penicillin: Ampicillin (AMP, 10 µg); 2th–4th generation cephalosporins: Cefoxitin (CX, 30 µg), Cefuroxime (CX, 30 µg), Ceftazidime (CFZ, 30 µg), Cefotaxime (CTX, 30 µg), Ceftriaxone (CRO, 30 µg), Cefepime (FEP, 30 µg); Monobactams: Aztreonam (ATM, 30 µg); β-lactam combination agents: Amoxicillin/Clavulanate (AMC, 20/10 µg), Ampicillin/Sulbactam (10/10 µg); Tetracyclines: Tetracycline (TE, 30 µg); Carbapenems: Imipenem (IMP, 10 µg), Meropenem (MEM, 10 µg), and Ertapenem (ETP, 10 µg). According to number of antibiotic categories, clinical isolates were classified as no multidrug resistant (NMDR, non-susceptible to less than 3 antibiotic categories), multidrug resistant (MDR, non-susceptible to at least 1 agent in 3 antimicrobial categories), extensively resistant (XDR, non-susceptible to at least 1 agent in all but two or fewer categories), or pandrug resistant (PDR, non-susceptible to all evaluated antimicrobial agents). Non-susceptible is defined as a clinical isolate which had resistant or intermediate resistant phenotype to an antimicrobial agent, according to Mayiorakos considerations [26].

2.9. Statistical Analysis

The results were analyzed using ANOVA Tukey's multiple comparisons test, Pearson correlation coefficient, and Fisher's exact test, using GraphPad Prims 6.04 software for Windows, GraphPad Software, La Jolla, CA, USA, www.graphpad.com, (accessed on 26 October 2021). The level of significance was considered as a p value $\leq$ 0.05. For Pearson correlation test, we statistically analyzed all genotypes, phenotypes, and phylogenetic groups against another; r values were obtained, and p value was confirmed with Fisher's exact test or Chi-square.

2.10. Ethic Statements

The protocol for this study was approved by the ethical committee from Universidad de Sonora (CEI-UNISON) (Registry number 07.2019, 12 March 2019).

3. Results

3.1. Clinical Characteristics of Adult Women with UTI

Ninety-eight urine samples were analyzed. Eighty-five were included in this study, whereas the remaining were obtained from men, children, or those who refused to give consent and were not included. Forty (47%) patients had UTI according to urine culture results.

The included patients (n = 85) average age was 47 years old, ranging from 19 to 80 years. No statistical significance was observed between average age of patients with UTI and without it (p < 0.05). Fifty-four (63%) had co-morbidities and UTI predisposing conditions, with diabetes, hypertension, hypothyroidism, renal failure, and previous diagnosis of UTI being the most frequent. Nevertheless, no statistically significant association of these conditions with UTI was observed. On the other hand, in urinalysis, statistically significant differences were observed for the higher prevalence of positive leukocyte esterase, pyuria, and bacteriuria in urine samples from patients with UTI vs. patients without UTI (Table 2a).

Table 2. Urinalysis, comorbidities, and urine culture results.

	(a) Included Patients' Groups (n = 85)			(b) Patients with UTI Caused by UPEC (n = 37)		
	With UTI n = 40 (%)	Without UTI n = 45 (%)	p	With Morphotype n = 24 (%)	Without Morphotype n = 13 (%)	p
Urinalysis						
pH:						
5.0–6.5	33 (83)	39 (87)	0.55	22 (92)	11 (85)	0.6
7.0–8.0	7 (17)	6 (13)		2 (8)	2 (15)	
LE:						
Positive	25 (63) *	12 (27)	0.002	16 (67)	7 (53)	0.49
Negative	15 (37)	33 (73)		8 (33)	6 (46)	
Pyuria:						
Positive (>5 WBCs/HPF)	31 (78) *	13 (29)	<0.0001	14 (58)	10 (85)	0.72
Negative (<5 WBCs/HPF)	9 (22)	32 (71)		10 (42)	4 (15)	
Bacteriuria:						
>2+	23 (58)	0 (0)	<0.0001	7 (29)	13 (100)	<0.0001
<2+	17 (42)	45 (100) *		17 (71) *	0 (0)	
Comorbidities						
Diabetes	11 (28)	12 (27)	>0.99	7 (29)	4 (31)	>0.99
Renal failure	3 (8)	3 (7)	>0.99	1 (4)	2 (15)	0.28
Hypertension	10 (25)	12 (27)	>0.99	5 (20)	3 (23)	>0.99
Diagnosed ITU	6 (15)	2 (4)	0.12	3 (13)	3 (23)	0.64
Vaginal infection	4 (10)	4 (9)	>0.99	0 (0) *	3 (23)	0.037
Pregnancy	3 (8)	1 (2)	0.33	2 (8)	1 (8)	>0.99
Hypothyroidism	1 (3)	5 (11)	0.2	0 (0)	1 (8)	0.35
Urine culture						
<100,000 CFU/mL	17 (43)	45 (100) *	<0.0001	17 (71)	-	<0.0001
>100,000 CFU/mL	20 (50)	0 (0)		7 (29)	13 (100)	

LE: Leucocyte esterase; WBCs/HPF: White blood cells per high power field. The higher prevalence of LE, pyuria, and bacteriuria in patients with UTI was significant, in comparison to the same prevalence in patients without UTI ($p < 0.05$). The higher prevalence of bacteriuria <2+ in urine sediments with bacterial morphotype than without it was significant ($p < 0.05$). p value was determined by Fisher's exact test. Values with statistical significance are indicated with *.

Twenty-five (62%) patients with UTI (n = 40) were symptomatic, with renal pain being the most frequent clinical symptom (73%). Fourteen of these patients (56%) showed lower urinary tract symptoms, dysuria being the most prevalent (100%). Other symptoms were fetid urine (12%) and urinary frequency (16%). More than one symptom was observed in 15 (60%) patients. On the other hand, 15 (38%) patients, with positive urine culture, were asymptomatic.

Additionally, twenty-eight (70%) of the patients with positive urine cultures reported recurrent UTI with two or more episodes each year. Ten (36%) of this patient's group were under antibiotic treatment, with Cotrimoxazole being the most implemented (30%).

3.2. Urine Cultures

Forty (49%) included urine samples (n = 85) were positive in urine culture. Monomicrobial cultures were obtained from 28 (70%) urine samples. The prevalence of uropathogens in monomicrobial cultures was *Escherichia coli* (89.2%), *Staphylococcus epidermidis* (3.5%), *Salmonella* spp. (3.5%), and *Citrobacter sedlakii* (3.5%). On the other hand, polymicrobial cultures were obtained from 12 (30%) of the analyzed urine samples, where *Escherichia coli* was found with other microorganisms in 9 (75%) samples. On MacConkey agar, three polymicrobial cultures with two different colonial morphologies (lactose positive and mucoid lactose positive) were observed, and both were identified as *E. coli*. The other microorganisms identified in polymicrobial cultures were *Buttiaxella agrestis*, *Moellerella wisconsensis, Citrobacter werkmanii*, and *Citrobacter gilenii*. Forty clinical isolates of *Escherichia coli* were obtained from all urine samples analyzed.

3.3. UPEC Morphotypes in Urine Sediment of Patients with UTI

UPEC morphotypes were observed in 24 (65%) of urine samples from patients with UTI caused by *E. coli* ($n = 37$). The most prevalent morphotypes were adherence (75%), IBC (54%), filamentous *E. coli* (25%), and biofilm (33%) (Figure 1). Morphotypes were frequently observed in combination (17/24 urine samples): Adherence+IBC (46%), Adherence+Biofilm (21%), Adherence+Filamentation (8%), Adherence+IBC+Filamentation (8%), and Adherence+IBC+Biofilm (8%). The etiologic agent of UTI in all urine samples with presence of morphotypes ($n = 24$) was *E. coli*; none of the urine samples with Gram positive bacteria showed evidence of morphotypes.

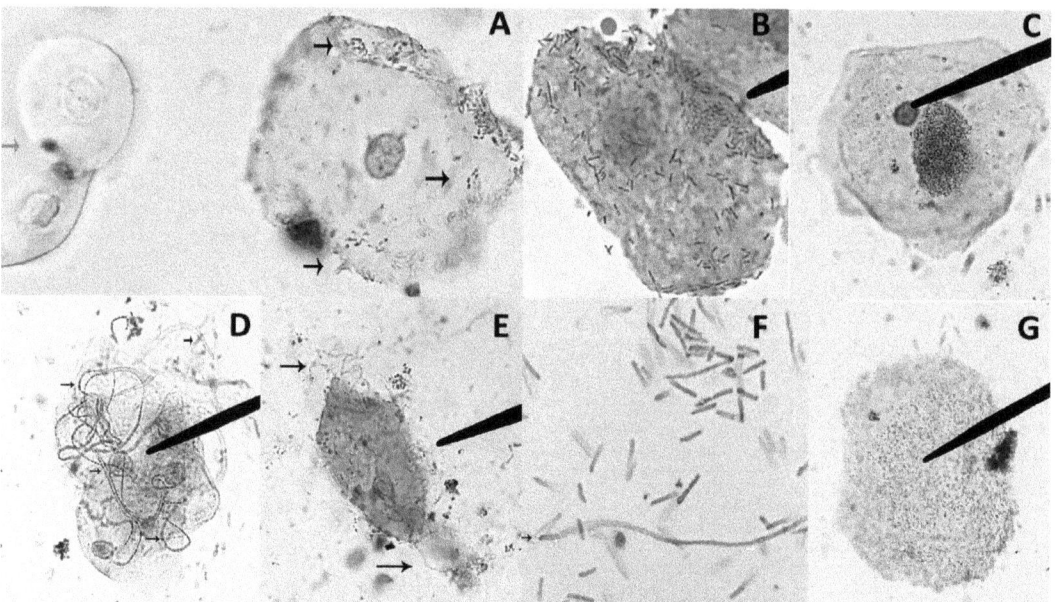

Figure 1. UPEC morphotypes observed in urinary sediment from patients with UTI. Light microscopic images of exfoliated uroepithelial cells and biofilm were stained with Sternheimer-Malbin dye. (**A**) Right: Vesical epithelial cell with bacterial adherence (black arrows) and left: renal epithelial cell (gray arrow) (40×). (**B**) Vesical epithelial cell with bacterial adherence (100×). (**C**) Vesical epithelial cells and Intracellular bacterial communities (40×). (**D**) Vesical epithelial cells and filamentous *E. coli* (40×). (**E**) Vesical epithelial cell with cytolysis and filamentous *E. coli* (black arrows) (40×). (**F**) Filamentous *E. coli* (black arrow) (100×). (**G**) Biofilm.

As expected, a higher prevalence of recurrent UTI episodes in patients with UPEC morphotypes in urinary sediments (71%) than in patients without them (46%) was observed; however, there was not statistical significance ($p > 0.05$). We also observed a higher prevalence of positive LE, and bacteriuria (>2+) in urine sediments with bacterial morphotypes than without it (Table 2b). Nevertheless, a significant difference was only found in the higher prevalence of bacteriuria (>2+) in urine samples with bacterial morphotype than without it ($p > 0.05$). It is important to note that urine cultures with a reduced number of CFU/mL were obtained more frequently from urine samples with bacterial morphotypes in comparison to those without ($p < 0.0001$) (Table 2b).

3.4. Prevalence of Virulence Associated Genes

The most prevalent virulence associated genes were *fimH* (100%), followed by *feoB* (98%) and *fliCD* (90%). A high prevalence of the S fimbriae subunit/F1C fimbriae chaperone gene (*sfaD/focC*) (73%), P pilus Adhesin gene (*papG-II*) (60%), capsule associated gene *kpsM* (60%), and vacuolating autotransporter toxin gene *vat* (48%) was also observed (Figure 2). Three common virulence profiles were observed in twenty-three (58%) clinical isolates (Table 3) and are related to both lower and upper UTI.

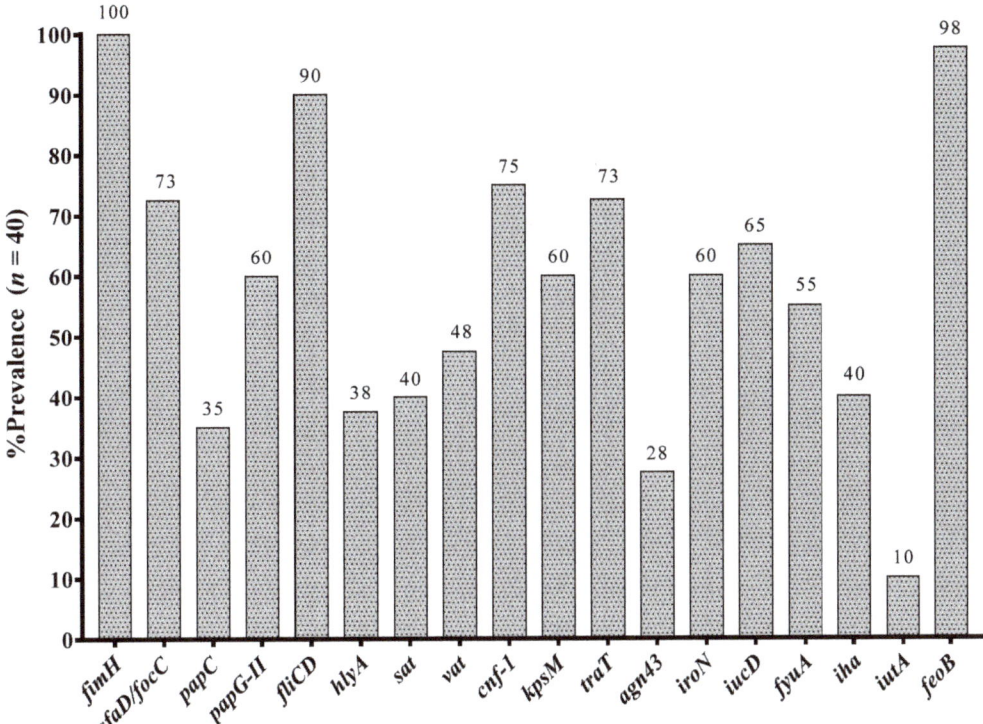

Figure 2. Prevalence of 18 virulence genes in analyzed clinical isolates of UPEC. ***fimH***: Fimbrial Adhesin of type 1 pilus; ***sfaD/focC***: S fimbriae minor subunit/F1C fimbriae chaperone; ***papC***: Type P pilus chaperone; ***papG-II***: Type P pilus Adhesin allele 2; ***fliCD***: Flagellin subunit/flagellar cap; ***hlyA***: α-hemolysin; ***sat***: Autotransporter secreted toxin; ***vat***: Vacuolating autotransporter toxin; ***cnf-1***: Necrotizing cytotoxic factor; ***kpsM***: Capsular variant; ***traT***: Serum resistance protein; ***agn43***: 43 antigen; ***iroN***: Salmochelin siderophore receptor; ***iucD***: Aerobactin; ***fyuA***: Yersiniabactin; ***iha***: Bifunctional enterobactin receptor/adhesin protein; ***iutA***: Ferric aerobactin receptor; ***feoB***: Ferrous iron transport protein B.

Table 3. Common virulence profile in analyzed clinical isolates of UPEC.

Virulence Profile	Clinical Isolates
fimH, feoB, fliCD, cnf-1, sfaD/focC	2,4–6,9–13,16,20,22–24,29,31,33–37,39–40
fimH, feoB, fliCD, cnf-1, sfaD/focC, traT, papG-II, kpsM	2,5,6,9,12,13,20,23,37
fimH. feoB, fliCD, cnf-1, sfaD/focC, traT, papG-II, kpsM, vat, sat	5,6,12,37

We compared the prevalence of virulence-associated genes between clinical isolates obtained from urine samples in which morphotype was observed vs. clinical isolates obtained from urine samples without morphotype. Statistical significance was only observed for the higher prevalence of *hlyA* (62%, $p = 0.04$), and *vat* (77%, $p = 0.01$) genes in UPEC isolates with IBC in urinary sediment versus those without morphotype (26% and 33%, respectively).

On the other hand, we observed that *E. coli* clinical isolates analyzed showed co-occurrence of some of the virulence-associated genes that we determined, and statistical significance was observed in all cases ($p < 0.05$). Interestingly, these genes are within pathogenicity islands (PAI) of prototypes UPEC strains such as *E. coli* 536, *E. coli* CFT073, *E. coli* J96, and *E. coli* UMN026. Table 4 shows genes for which a positive correlation and statistical significance was observed.

Table 4. Co-occurrence of virulence genes related with PAI in clinical isolates of UPEC.

Gene	% ($n = 40$)	r	p	Reported PAI [a]
			papG-II:	PAI I, IICFT073, PAI I-V536, PAI I-IIJ96
papC	32.5	0.49	0.001	PAI I-IICFT073
vat	40	0.47	0.002	Not named PAI Ec222
iroN	45	0.38	0.017	PAI III536
fyuA	42.5	0.39	0.012	PAI IICFT073, PAI III, IV536
sfaD/focC	72.5	0.54	<0.001	PAI I, IICFT073, PAI I-IVJ96, PAI I-IIJ96, PAI I-III536
			papC:	PAI IICFT073
iroN	30	0.38	0.0141	PAI III536
fyuA	30	0.45	0.003	PAI IICFT073, PAI III, IV536
			sat:	PAI IICFT073
vat	27.5	0.35	0.028	Not named PAI Ec222
iroN	35	0.46	0.002	PAI III536
fyuA	35	0.53	<0.001	PAI IICFT073, PAI III, IV536
kpsM	32.5	0.35	0.02	PAI V536
iucD	35	0.39	0.01	PAI IICFT073, PAI III-IV536, Not named PAI UMN026
			hlyA:	PAI ICFT073, PAI I-II536, PAI I-IIJ96
kpsM	35	0.53	<0.001	PAI V536
cnf-1	35	0.33	0.04	PAI IIJ96
			vat:	Not named PAI Ec222
cnf-1	42.5	0.32	0.05	PAI IIJ96
			cnf-1:	PAI IIJ96
iha	37.5	0.35	0.025	PAI I, IICFT073, PAI I-IVJ96, PAI I-IIJ96, PAI I-II536
KpsM	52.5	0.35	0.025	PAI V536
			iroN:	PAI III536
fyuA	47.5	0.59	<0.001	PAI IICFT073, PAI III, IV536

Statistical significance and correlation value (r) was obtained with Pearson correlation coefficient. For Pearson correlation test, we statistically analyzed all genotypes, phenotypes, and phylogenetic groups against another; r values were obtained and p value was confirmed with Fisher's exact test or Chi-square. Correlation is significant at 0.01 level (2-tailed). [a]: Accession link to Pathogenicity Island Database (PAI DB) *E. coli* Pathogenicity Island http://www.paidb.re.kr/browse_pais.php?m=p&SPC=Escherichia%20coli (accessed on 26 October 2021).

3.5. Virulence Phenotypes of Clinical Isolates of UPEC

The prevalence of some of the most important virulence phenotypes of UPEC was investigated. We found that 98% of clinical isolates were motile, 70% were capsule producers, and only 5% produced the hemolysis phenotype. We tried to identify relationships between genotypes vs. these virulence phenotypes; however, only a statistically significant association between the higher prevalence of *kpsM* ($p = 0.0367$) and *iha* ($x^2 = 0.048$) genes in capsule-producing isolates was observed.

All clinical isolates were biofilm producers (100%), but only 68% were strong biofilm producers (Figure 3). Comparing the prevalence of virulence genes in each biofilm producer group, a significant difference was observed only in the higher prevalence of *iucD* ($p = 0.03$) and *papC* ($p = 0.05$) genes in the strong biofilm producers.

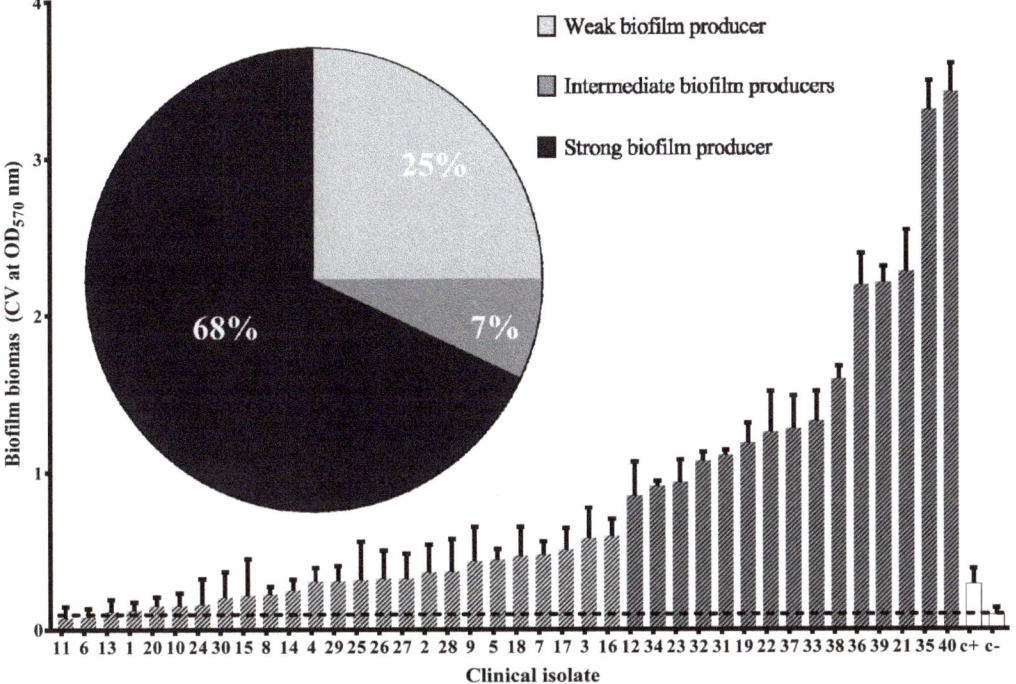

Figure 3. Biofilm production in clinical isolates of UPEC. The dotted line is at the level of the result obtained for the negative control. The biofilm biomass is expressed as the average OD at 570 nm of five independent experiments, error bars show standard deviation (SD). +C: Positive control (*Escherichia coli* 25922); -C: Negative control (sterile Mueller-Hinton Broth.). Dark bars show the stronger biofilm producers with the most statistical significance ($p < 0.05$) (Two-way ANOVA, Tukey's multiple comparisons test), white bars show the implemented controls. Pie chart at the top shows the percentage of weak, intermediate, and strong biofilm forming UPEC clinical isolates.

For adherence assay, twenty clinical isolates were selected according to their virulence profile and phylogenetic groups. Twenty-five percent of selected isolates were low adherent to HeLa cells, 15% were classified as moderately adherent, and 60% were strongly adherent. Fifteen (75%) of selected UPEC were more adherent than positive control (*E. coli* EDL 933) ($p = 0.0001$) (Figure 4). Interestingly, UPEC 12 was the most adherent and virulent isolate with 16/18 virulence associated genes.

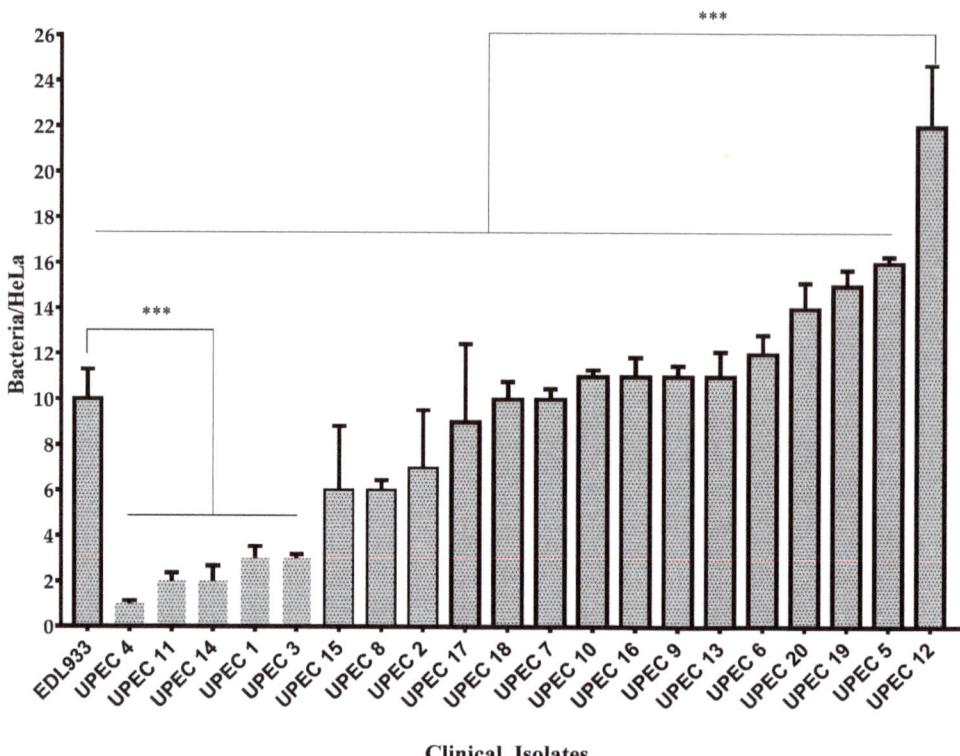

Figure 4. Adherence assay for UPEC clinical isolates. ***: $p = 0.0001$. One way ANOVA Tukey's multiple comparisons test. Adherence groups are shown in the graph. Bars with thick line: strongly adherent group; bars with thin line: moderately adherent group; bars without line: low adherent group. Total HeLa cells and adherent bacteria were counted in 10 fields at 40X objective. The results are expressed as the average number of adherent bacteria from three independent experiments. Error bars show standard error of the mean (SEM).

Positive correlation between strongly adherent UPEC with a higher prevalence of *papC* gene ($r = 0.471$, $p = 0.036$) was observed. No statistical significance between adherence groups, biofilm formation groups, phylogenetic groups, and UPEC morphotypes in urine was found ($p > 0.05$).

3.6. Antibiotic Resistance Phenotypes

Obtained clinical isolates showed a higher resistance to antibiotics of the β-lactam family, mainly ampicillin (80%), second and third generation cephalosporins: Cefuroxime (95%), Cefotaxime (83%), and the inhibitor combined β-lactamic: Amoxicillin/Clavulanate (80%). High resistance was also observed for aminoglycosides: Amikacin (60%) and Gentamicin (73%) (Figure 5). On the other hand, the isolates were predominantly sensitive to nitrofurantoin, one of the most widely used antibiotics in the treatment of UTI. According to Magyorakos criteria, only 7.5% of clinical isolates were not multidrug resistant (NMDR), while 85% were multidrug resistant (MDR), and 7.5% were classified as extremely resistant (XDR). Additionally, one clinical isolate was sensitive for all tested antibiotics. Distribution of antibiotic resistant in all clinical isolates is shown in Supplementary Material Table S2. Most common resistance profile was AMK, GM, AMP, CFX, CTX, and AMC, found in 17 (43%) clinical isolates. No statistical significance was observed between biofilm producers groups, bacterial morphotypes, and antibiotic resistance [26].

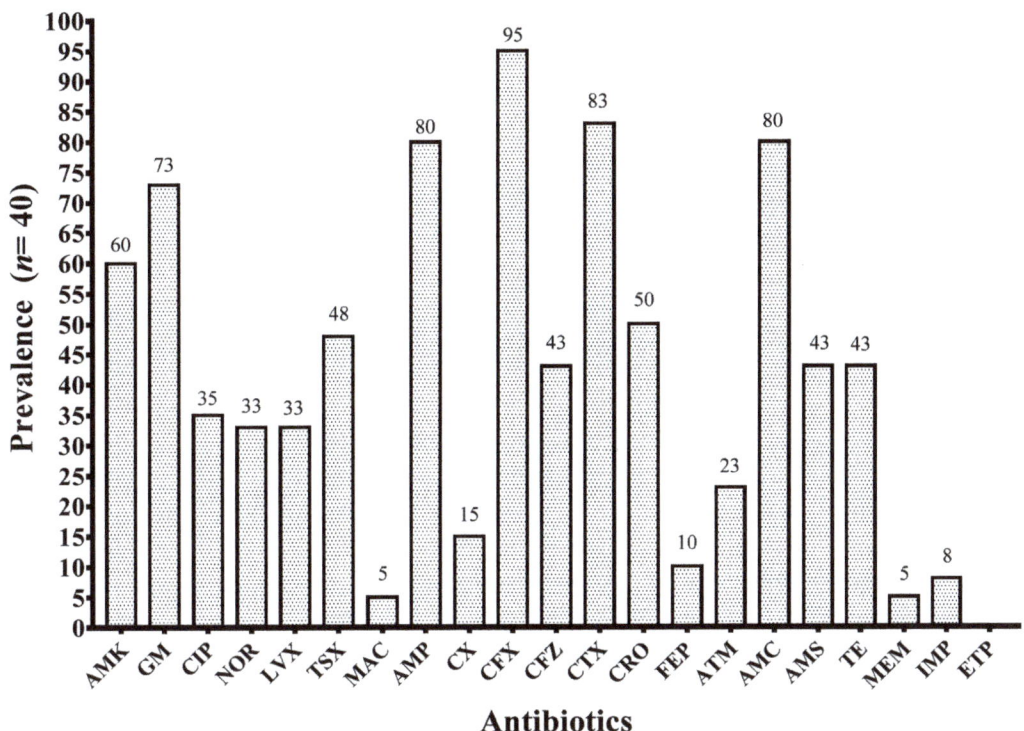

Figure 5. Antibiotic resistance prevalence. **AMK**: Amikacin; **GM**: Gentamicin; **CIP**: Ciprofloxacin; **NOR**: Norfloxacin; **LVX**: Levofloxacin; **TSX**: Cotrimoxazole; **MAC**: Nitrofurantoin; **AMP**: Ampicillin; **CX**: Cefoxitin; **CFX**: Cefuroxime; **CFZ**: Ceftazidime; **CTX**: Cefotaxime; **CRO**: Ceftriaxone; **FEP**: Cefepime; **ATM**: Aztreonam; **AMC**: Amoxicillin/Clavulanate; **AMS**: Ampicillin/Sulbactam; **TE**: Tetracyclin; **MEM**: Meropenem; **IMP**: Imipenem; **ETP**: Ertapenem.

3.7. Phylogenetic Groups of Obtained Clinical Isolates

The prevalent phylogenetic group of the bacterial population studied was B2 (27.5%), followed by B1 (22.5%), E (15%), and C (10%). Twenty-five percent of the clinical isolates belonged to unknown phylogenetic groups (NT). No isolates belonging to groups A, D, and F were observed.

According to the mean of virulence genes in each phylogenetic group, more virulent UPEC isolates belong to B2 phylogenetic group. However, statistical significance was observed only in the higher mean of virulence of B2 vs. B1 and NT phylogenetic groups (Figure 6). We also observed that the prevalence of specific virulence genes was different between phylogenetic groups. In this sense, *papC*, *iroN*, and *fyuA*, which are genes related to highly pathogenic *E. coli*, were most prevalent in isolates from B2 phylogenetic group (Table 5).

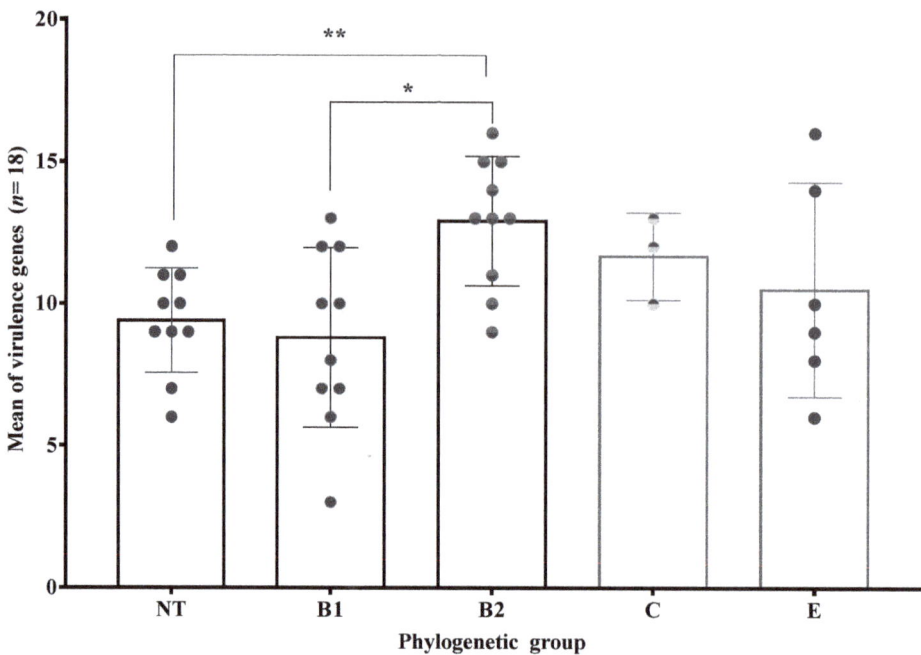

Figure 6. Mean of virulence by phylogenetic groups. **: $p = 0.01$; *: $p = 0.04$. One way ANOVA Tukey's multiple comparisons test. Error bars show standard deviation (SD) and each gray dot represent clinical isolates of specific phylogenetic group.

Table 5. Virulence genes distribution between phylogenetic groups of UPEC clinical isolates.

Gene	NT $n = 10$ (%)	p	B1 $n = 10$ (%)	p	B2 $n = 11$ (%)	p	C $n = 3$ (%)	p	E $n = 6$ (%)	p	Total $n = 40$ (%)
fimH	10 (100)	1	10 (100)	1	11 (100)	1	3 (100)	1	6 (100)	1	14 (35)
papC	2 (20)	0.7	2 (20)	0.7	7 (64)	0.02	0 (0)	0.53	3 (50)	0.64	40 (100)
papG-II	6 (60)	1	4 (40)	0.15	9 (82)	0.13	3 (100)	0.26	2 (33)	0.19	29 (73)
sfaD/focC	8 (80)	0.69	9 (90)	0.23	7 (64)	0.45	3 (100)	0.54	2 (33)	0.03	24 (60)
fliCD	10 (100)	0.55	9 (90)	1	10 (91)	1	3 (100)	1	4 (67)	0.09	36 (90)
cnf-1	8 (80)	1	7 (70)	0.68	9 (82)	0.69	2 (67)	1	4 (67)	0.62	16 (40)
vat	4 (40)	0.72	4 (40)	0.72	6 (55)	0.72	2 (67)	0.59	3 (50)	1	15 (38)
sat	3 (30)	0.71	1 (10)	0.06	7 (64)	0.08	2 (67)	0.55	3 (50)	0.66	24 (60)
hlyA	4 (40)	1	4 (40)	1	6 (55)	0.27	0 (0)	0.27	1 (17)	0.38	19 (48)
feoB	10 (100)	1	9 (90)	1	11 (100)	1	3 (100)	1	6 (100)	1	30 (75)
iucD	4 (40)	0.12	5 (50)	0.27	9 (82)	0.26	2 (67)	1	6 (100)	0.07	29 (73)
iroN	4 (40)	0.15	3 (30)	0.05	10 (91)	0.02	3 (100)	0.26	4 (67)	1	11 (28)
fyuA	4 (40)	0.3	1 (10)	0.002	11 (100)	0.0003	2 (67)	0.99	4 (67)	0.67	24 (60)
iha	1 (10)	0.03	4 (40)	1	6 (55)	0.29	2 (67)	0.55	3 (50)	0.66	26 (65)
iutA	0 (0)	0.55	3 (30)	0.71	9 (82)	1	0 (0)	1	0 (0)	1	22 (55)
traT	9 (90)	0.23	4 (40)	0.01	8 (73)	1	2 (67)	1	6 (100)	0.16	16 (40)
kpsM	5 (50)	0.48	5 (50)	0.48	9 (82)	0.14	1 (33)	0.55	4 (67)	0.63	4 (10)
agn43	2 (20)	0.69	4 (40)	0.41	1 (9)	0.23	2 (67)	0.17	2 (33)	1	39 (98)

The p values were calculated with Fisher Exact Test comparing the prevalence of the virulence gene in each phylogenetic group with all other combined groups. Values significantly higher than the other groups are showed in red boxes, while values significantly lower than the other groups are shown in purple boxes.

Analyzing results of virulence phenotypes, we observed a positive correlation between phylogenetic group B2 and hemolysis ($r = 0.37$, $p = 0.017$) and a negative correlation between phylogroup NT and capsule production ($r = -0.38$, $p = 0.016$). In adherence assays, a negative correlation between high adherent bacteria and phylogenetic group C was observed. No statistically significant association between biofilm producers' groups, morphotypes in urine sediment, and phylogenetic group was found.

Regarding antibiotic resistance, a statistically significant difference was only observed in the higher number of antibiotics to which clinical isolates of phylogenetic group B1 showed resistance compared to those belonging to phylogenetic group NT (Figure 7).

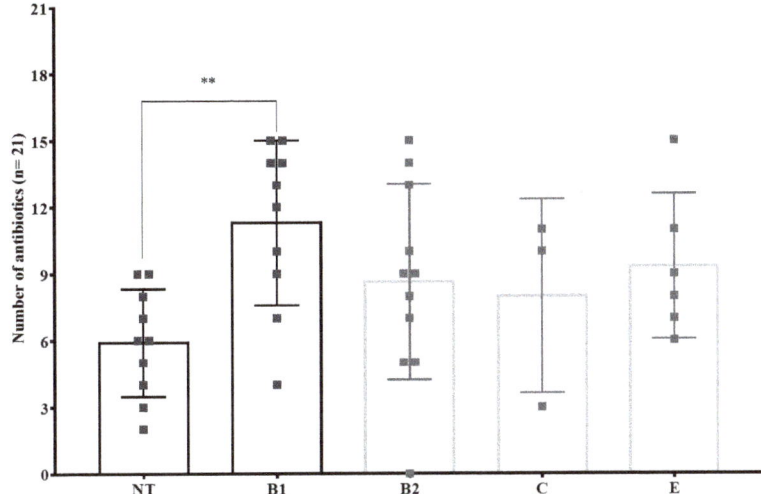

Figure 7. Mean of antibiotic resistance by phylogenetic groups. **: $p = 0.01$. One way ANOVA Tukey's multiple comparisons test. Error bars show standard deviation (SD) and each gray square represent clinical isolates of specific phylogenetic group.

4. Discussion

In this study, the prevalence of bacterial morphotypes in urine sediments, virulence associated genes, virulence phenotypes, and phylogenetic groups of UPEC were investigated.

In polymicrobial cultures, together with *Escherichia coli*, we found some atypical urinary tract pathogens. These were *Moellerella wisconsensis* and *Buttiaxella agrestis*, which are microorganisms commonly reported in infectious processes in other animal species, such as dogs or cats, and only in a few reports as causative agents of human infections after surgical procedures or in immunosuppressed patients [27–29]. In this sense, it is important to mention that in this work both isolates were obtained from diabetic patients that expressed having at least one previous UTI episode. It is reported that diabetic patients have four times more probability of developing infectious diseases, including UTI, and the etiology of these infections include atypical pathogens, this being a possible explication for our results [30–32]. Interestingly, to our knowledge, this is the first report of *Butiaxella agrestis* and *Moellerella wisconsensis* isolated from UTI in México.

Nowadays polymicrobial infections have gained importance due to their probable association with therapeutic failures and horizontal gene transfer between pathogens [33,34]. In this sense, in polymicrobial cultures, we observed the presence of some species of the genus *Citrobacter*, such as *Citrobacter sedlakii*, *Citrobacter gillenii*, and *Citrobacter werckmanii*. These microorganisms are considered emerging pathogens in several infectious processes including urinary tract infections [35,36], and are also resistant to antibiotics used as treatment of UTI, mainly Cotrimoxazole, quinolones, and β-lactam antibiotics [27–29,36–39].

Therefore, it would be interesting to investigate and compare the resistance characteristics of these microorganisms with those of *E. coli* obtained from the same urine sample.

The presence of bacterial morphotypes in urine is important due to their association with immune evasion and antibiotic resistance. In this regard, we found that 65% of the *E. coli* isolates were obtained from urines samples with morphotypes. These results are higher than those reported by Robino et al. in 2013 and 2014 [10,40], who found morphotypes in only 22.6% of the analyzed urine samples. Interestingly, 17 (71%) of the urine samples that showed morphotypes were negative in urine culture. However, by applying vortex to release the intracellular bacteria, the CFU/mL counts increased, and the urine cultures were positives (>100,000 CFU/mL). Therefore, when IBC are observed, we suggest the implementation of bacterial releasing methods to reduce false negatives in urine cultures. On the other hand, in seven of the urine samples with morphotype, positive urine cultures were obtained despite the presence of IBC. This could be explained by the number of extracellular bacteria present in the sample, because part of the process of maturation of the IBC leads to the release of bacteria into the extracellular medium.

We also observed that bacterial morphotypes were more frequent in urine sediments from patients with recurrent UTI episodes than patients without it. This is in accordance with the reported by Robino, Rosen, and Martinez-Figueroa [11,17,40]. These results suggest that the method used in the clinical diagnosis of UTI needs to be modified, the search for these UPEC morphotypes in urinary sediment must be done routinely to avoid misdiagnosis, and Sternheimer-Malbin dye could be implemented for detection of these bacterial morphotypes. In addition to IBC and filamentous bacteria in urinary sediment, we considered it important to report the presence of bacterial adherence to bladder cells and biofilms in urinary sediment, since both play a significant role in the pathogenic mechanism of UPEC and could be involved in the persistence of this pathogen in the urinary tract. To our knowledge, this is the first report of prevalence of UPEC bacterial morphotypes in urinary sediment of Mexican population.

When analyzing the clinical data collected from the patients, we found that 30% of the women with recurrent UTI episodes were undergoing or had completed treatment with Cotrimoxazole. In Mexico, there are several reports demonstrating the high resistance of clinical isolates of UPEC to this antimicrobial agent which has led to considering its therapeutic efficacy. However, it would be important to continue with research focused on the determination of local susceptibility profiles for the antibiotics included in the basic treatment for UTI in Mexico, since it is known that resistance profiles can differ depending on the geographic area [14,16,41–45].

Antimicrobial resistance is currently a challenge in health because therapeutic options are reduced. In this study we found that the clinical isolates obtained were predominantly multidrug resistant (93%) and showed a high resistance to antibiotics implemented in the basic treatment of UTI, mainly aminoglycosides, β-lactams, and cotrimoxazole. These results are in agreement with those reported in previous studies [14,16] in Mexico, which highlights the urgent need to search for therapeutic alternatives for the treatment of UTI.

Regarding virulence, we observed that all clinical isolates carried the *fimH* gene. Our results are similar to those reported in previous works in Peru and Ethiopia, where a prevalence of 98% and 82% for *fimH* in clinical isolates of UPEC was reported [46,47]. In Mexico, Miranda-Estrada et al. 2017; Morales-Espinosa et al. 2016, López-Banda. 2014, and Ballesteros-Monrreal et al. 2020 reported a prevalence of 96%, 100%, 86%, and 100%, respectively, for this Adhesin [14,15,48,49]. This was not unexpected since *fimH* is crucial in the development of UPEC uropathogenic mechanism, including IBC formation.

Among the identified genes associated with pyelonephritis, the gene associated with flagellum (*fliCD*) was the most prevalent (90%). This prevalence is higher than the reported in previous studies conducted by Tabasi et al., 2016 in Iran and Qingqing et al., 2017 in China where a prevalence of 68% and 15%, respectively, was observed [50,51]. In this regard, in Mexico there is scarce evidence concerning the prevalence of this gene in clinical isolates of UPEC; however, in recent reports by Ordaz-López in Mexico City and

Ballesteros-Monrreal in the state of Puebla, the *fliC* gene has been observed in 25% and 30%, respectively [14,52]. On the other hand, the *papG-II* gene which codify for type P pilus Adhesin was also highly prevalent (60%). These results are different to those reported in other work in Mexico by Bravata-Alcantara and Luna-Pineda, who reported a prevalence of 21.5% and 15.4%, respectively [53,54]. Our results suggest that clinical isolates from the State of Sonora have a greater potential to cause upper UTIs compared to other Mexican states. Additionally, despite the scarce existing information, the reports available in Mexico show a higher prevalence of these genes in our country compared to others [55,56].

Similarly, a high prevalence of the *sfaD/focC* gene was also observed (73%), which is associated with both pili S and pili F1C. This gene is of interest because it is not only associated with pyelonephritis, but also meningitis and septicemia in adults [57]. Additionally, we observed that 72.5% of the clinical isolates that presented the *sfaD/focC* gene also presented the *papG-II* gene, associated with type P pili. This could be explained by the fact that both genes are harbored within the pathogenicity island (PAI) III of *Escherichia coli* 536 [58]. Interestingly, in addition to *sfaD/focC* and *papG-II* a high prevalence of clinical isolates with co-occurrence of virulence genes reported in PAI was observed (Table 4). Presence of PAIs could indicate a high pathogenic potential, so it would be interesting to determine in the future the presence of these genetic elements in our clinical isolates.

We also observed a considerable prevalence of the genes *kpsM* (60%), *sat* (40%), and *hlyA* (38%). These results are similar to those previously reported in Mexico [15,57,59]. The *kpsM* gene is associated with capsule production, and it is known that capsules may contribute to immune evasion, mainly in serum resistance, phagocytosis, and resistance to death by neutrophils and monocytes [7,60]. On the other hand, the *sat* and *hlyA* are toxigenicity associated genes involved mainly in upper UTI. The Sat protein has been reported as a vacuolating cytotoxin in cultured mammalian bladder and kidney cells [61]. While HlyA protein is a toxin with cytolytic effect, it is also involved in iron acquisition, since iron can be released from damaged cells [62], which is subsequently captured by siderophores produced by UPEC. Additionally, this protein can act as an immunomodulator at sublytic concentrations favoring UPEC immune evasion, even during bacteriemia [9,63,64]. Despite the high prevalence of the *hlyA* gene, we only observed hemolysis phenotype in 5% of the analyzed clinical isolates. These results are similar to those previously reported by our work group, where a prevalence of the gene in clinical isolates from Sonora of 38–56% and a coincidence with the hemolysis phenotype of 12–16% were observed [14]. The higher prevalence of the *hlyA* gene compared to its respective phenotype could be explained by the fact that the HlyA protein is the immature toxin, which requires a prior acetylation step to generate its lytic effect.

The most common phenotype observed was biofilm production (100%); 60% of the clinical isolates were strong biofilm producers. This phenotype is important since it is associated with antimicrobial resistance. When analyzing the prevalence of each of the virulence-associated genes among biofilm-producing groups, we observed a higher prevalence of the *iucD* and *papC* genes in the strong biofilm producers. Interestingly, neither of the aforementioned genes are directly implicated in biofilm formation, but both have been reported to be associated with genomic islands. Similar results were found in adherence phenotypes, where a positive correlation was found between the *papC* gene and the strong adherence group; this gene was not observed in any of the isolates that presented weak or medium adherence. *papC* encodes for the helper chaperone protein of the pyelonephritis-associated pili and is not directly associated with the adherence phenotype, so, as with biofilm production, it is probably that another gene associated with the same pathogenicity island in which *papC* or *iucD* are harbored is directly involved with these phenotypes.

The prevalence of phylogenetic groups in the obtained isolates was also examined. Interestingly, a high prevalence of clinical isolates that could not be phylogenetically classified (25%) was observed, which could indicate the presence of new phylogenetic groups in Sonora, and these results are in accordance with those previously reported by our work group in Puebla and Sonora [14].

It is thought that the most pathogenic isolates are clustered in phylogenetic groups B2 and D, while the most resistant and commensal isolates are located in groups A and B1. Comparing the average of virulence associated genes by phylogenetic group, we observed statistically significant differences between the highest number of virulence genes in phylogroup B2 compared to phylogroup B1 and non-typeable (NT), but not with phylogroups C and E. However, no statistically significant difference was found between the average number of virulence genes present in phylogroups B1, NT, C, and E. Similar results were observed in antibiotic resistant. Clinical isolates classified as B1 were more resistant than NT ($p < 0.05$), but no than the phylogroups B2, C, and E. This could suggest that virulence and antibiotic resistance are not restricted to the specifics phylogenetics groups.

In summary, we observed that all clinical isolates presented the *fimH* gene, which is indicative of pathogens that have the capacity to cause lower urinary tract infections. In addition, 65% of the UPEC with the *fimH* gene presented bacterial morphotypes in urinary sediment, indicating that they are bacteria with the ability to cause lower UTI and internalize, forming IBC or bacterial filaments, which allow them to avoid the host immune response, resist the effects of antimicrobial treatments, and persist in the urinary tract leading to recurrent episodes of UTI. Seventy-three percent of clinical isolates also present the *fliCD* gene or the motile phenotype and any of the *papG-II*, *papC*, or *sfaD/focC* genes that are related to renal adherence; therefore, these pathogens have the capacity to cause both lower UTI and upper UTI. Finally, a high percent of the obtained isolates presented each of the characteristics described above together with the α-hemolysin genes or the secreted autotransporter toxin (*sat*) as well as the gene *kpsM* or capsule phenotype, suggesting highly pathogenic UPEC which are potentially capable of causing both types of UTI, evading the host immune system, resisting antibiotic treatment, persisting in the urinary tract, and causing recurrent UTI. Additionally, these bacteria have potential to induce renal damage, and gain access to the bloodstream and cause bacteremia.

5. Conclusions

In conclusion, UPEC's clinical isolates obtained from adult women in Sonora were MDR and had a high pathogenic potential to cause lower and upper UTI. In Mexico, the actual prevalence of UPEC bacterial morphotypes in urinary sediment is unknown. However, the available evidence indicates that it is a common phenomenon in the Mexican population and is associated not only with recurrence of UTI but also with false negatives in urine culture, which considerably delays the treatment of the infectious process and could lead to more serious complications. Therefore, diagnostic methods in the clinical laboratory should include the search for these morphotypes in urinalysis.

Supplementary Materials: The following are available online at https://www.mdpi.com/article/10.3390/microorganisms9112381/s1, Table S1: Genes and phenotype traits from the strains selected for adherence assays. Table S2: Antibiotic resistance distribution in obtained clinical isolates of UPEC.

Author Contributions: M.G.B.-M.: conceptualization, methodology, formal analysis, investigation, and writing—original draft; M.M.P.A.-H.: writing—review and editing and resources; E.B.-V.: writing—review and editing and resources; J.J.: writing—review and editing and resources; M.L.Á.-A.: writing—review and editing and resources; P.T.: writing—review and editing and resources; R.D.l.R.-L.: writing—review and editing and resources; E.B.-M.: writing—review and editing, resources, project administration, and supervision; D.V.: writing—review and editing, resources, project administration, and supervision. All authors have read and agreed to the published version of the manuscript.

Funding: This research was funded by Departamento de ciencias Químico-Biológicas y Agropecuarias, and División de Ciencias e Ingenierías from Universidad de Sonora, Unidad Regional Norte (UNISON URN).

Institutional Review Board Statement: The study was conducted according to the guidelines of the Declaration of Helsinki, and approved by the Institutional Ethics Committee of Universidad de Sonora (CEI-UNISON) (Registry number 07.2019. 12 March 2019).

Informed Consent Statement: Informed consent was obtained from all subjects involved in the study.

Acknowledgments: The authors are pleased to acknowledge the Departamento de ciencias Químico-Biológicas y Agropecuarias, and División de Ciencias e Ingenierías from Universidad de Sonora. Thanks to Pablo Mendez-Pfeiffer from Universidad de Sonora for proofreading the manuscript. Manuel G. Ballesteros-Monrreal had a CONACYT Fellowship during the performance of this work (Scholarship No. 617232).

Conflicts of Interest: The authors declare no conflict of interest.

References

1. Secretaría de Salud Boletín de Semana Epidemiológica 53. Available online: https://www.gob.mx/salud/acciones-y-programas/historico-boletin-epidemiologico (accessed on 12 January 2021).
2. Secretaría de Salud Boletín de Semana Epidemiológica 52. Available online: https://www.gob.mx/salud/acciones-y-programas/historico-boletin-epidemiologico (accessed on 12 January 2021).
3. Foxman, B. The epidemiology of urinary tract infection. *Nat. Rev. Urol.* **2010**, *7*, 653–660. [CrossRef] [PubMed]
4. Flores-Mireles, A.L.; Walker, J.N.; Caparon, M.; Hultgren, S.J. Urinary tract infections: Epidemiology, mechanisms of infection and treatment options. *Nat. Rev. Microbiol.* **2015**, *13*, 269–284. [CrossRef] [PubMed]
5. Morimoto, Y.; Minamino, T. Structure and Function of the Bi-Directional Bacterial Flagellar Motor. *Biomolecules* **2014**, *4*, 217–234. [CrossRef] [PubMed]
6. Roberts, J.A.; Marklund, B.I.; Ilver, D.; Haslam, D.; Kaack, M.B.; Baskin, G.; Louis, M.; Mollby, R.; Winberg, J.; Normark, S. The Gal(alpha 1-4)Gal-specific tip adhesin of Escherichia coli P-fimbriae is needed for pyelonephritis to occur in the normal urinary tract. *Proc. Natl. Acad. Sci. USA* **1994**, *91*, 11889–11893. [CrossRef]
7. Livorsi, D.J.; Stenehjem, E.; Stephens, D.S. Virulence Factors of Gram- Negative Bacteria in Sepsis with a Focus on Neisseria meningitidis. *Contrib Microbiol* **2011**, *17*, 31–47.
8. González, M.J.; Da Cunda, P.; Notejane, M.; Zunino, P.; Scavone, P.; Robino, L. Fosfomycin tromethamine activity on biofilm and intracellular bacterial communities produced by uropathogenic Escherichia coli isolated from patients with urinary tract infection. *Pathog. Dis.* **2019**, *77*, ftz022. [CrossRef]
9. Olson, P.; Hunstad, D. Subversion of Host Innate Immunity by Uropathogenic Escherichia coli. *Pathogens* **2016**, *5*, 2. [CrossRef]
10. Robino, L.; Scavone, P.; Araujo, L.; Algorta, G.; Zunino, P.; Pírez, M.C.; Vignoli, R. Intracellular bacteria in the pathogenesis of escherichia coli urinary tract infection in children. *Clin. Infect. Dis.* **2014**, *59*, e158–e164. [CrossRef]
11. Rosen, D.A.; Hooton, T.M.; Stamm, W.E.; Humphrey, P.A.; Hultgren, S.J. Detection of intracellular bacterial communities in human urinary tract infection. *PLoS Med.* **2007**, *4*, 1949–1958. [CrossRef]
12. Clermont, O.; Bonacorsi, S.; Bingen, E. Rapid and simple determination of the Escherichia coli phylogenetic group. *Appl. Environ. Microbiol.* **2000**, *66*, 4555–4558. [CrossRef]
13. Clermont, O.; Christenson, J.K.; Denamur, E.; Gordon, D.M. The Clermont Escherichia coli phylo-typing method revisited: Improvement of specificity and detection of new phylo-groups. *Environ. Microbiol. Rep.* **2013**, *5*, 58–65. [CrossRef] [PubMed]
14. Ballesteros-Monrreal, M.G.; Arenas-Hernández, M.M.P.; Enciso-Martínez, Y.; Martinez de la Peña, C.F.; Rocha-Gracia, R.d.C.; Lozano-Zarain, P.; Navarro-Ocaña, A.; Martínez-Laguna, Y.; de la Rosa-López, R. Virulence and Resistance Determinants of Uropathogenic Escherichia coli Strains Isolated from Pregnant and Non-Pregnant Women from Two States in Mexico. *Infect. Drug Resist.* **2020**, *13*, 295–310. [CrossRef] [PubMed]
15. Miranda-Estrada, L.I.; Ruíz-Rosas, M.; Molina-López, J.; Parra-Rojas, I.; González-Villalobos, E.; Castro-Alarcón, N. Relación entre factores de virulencia, resistencia a antibióticos y los grupos filogenéticos de Escherichia coli uropatógena en dos localidades de México. *Enferm. Infecc. Microbiol. Clin.* **2017**, *35*, 426–433. [CrossRef] [PubMed]
16. Iranpour, D.; Hassanpour, M.; Ansari, H.; Tajbakhsh, S.; Khamisipour, G.; Najafi, A. Phylogenetic Groups of Escherichia coli Strains from Patients with Urinary Tract Infection in Iran Based on the New Clermont Phylotyping Method. *Biomed Res. Int.* **2015**, *2015*, 1–7. [CrossRef]
17. Martínez-Figueroa, C.; Cortés-Sarabia, K.; Del Carmen Alarcón-Romero, L.; Catalán-Nájera, H.G.; Martínez-Alarcón, M.; Vences-Velázquez, A. Observation of intracellular bacterial communities in urinary sediment using brightfield microscopy; A case report. *BMC Urol.* **2020**. [CrossRef]
18. KASS, E.H. Pyelonephritis and Bacteriuria. *Ann. Intern. Med.* **1962**, *56*, 46. [CrossRef]
19. Sambrook, J. *Molecular Cloning: A Laboratory Manual*; Cold Spring Harbor: New York, NY, USA, 2012; Volume 33, ISBN 9781936113415.
20. Walker, D.I.; McQuillan, J.; Taiwo, M.; Parks, R.; Stenton, C.A.; Morgan, H.; Mowlem, M.C.; Lees, D.N. A highly specific Escherichia coli qPCR and its comparison with existing methods for environmental waters. *Water Res.* **2017**, *126*, 101–110. [CrossRef]

21. Christensen, G.D.; Simpson, W.A.; Younger, J.J.; Baddour, L.M.; Barrett, F.F.; Melton, D.M.; Beachey, E.H. Adherence of coagulase-negative staphylococci to plastic tissue culture plates: A quantitative model for the adherence of staphylococci to medical devices. *J. Clin. Microbiol.* **1985**, *22*, 996–1006. [CrossRef]
22. Luna, V.A.; Peak, K.K.; Veguilla, W.O.; Reeves, F.; Heberlein-Larson, L.; Cannons, A.C.; Amuso, P.; Cattani, J. Use of Two Selective Media and a Broth Motility Test Can Aid in Identification or Exclusion of Bacillus anthracis. *J. Clin. Microbiol.* **2005**, *43*, 4336–4341. [CrossRef]
23. Anthony, E.E. a Note on Capsule Staining. *Science* **1931**, *73*, 319–320. [CrossRef]
24. Barrios-Villa, E.; Cortés-Cortés, G.; Lozano-Zaraín, P.; de la Paz Arenas-Hernández, M.M.; Martínez de la Peña, C.F.; Martínez-Laguna, Y.; Torres, C.; Rocha-Gracia, R.D.C. Adherent/invasive Escherichia coli (AIEC) isolates from asymptomatic people: New E. coli ST131 O25:H4/H30-Rx virotypes. *Ann. Clin. Microbiol. Antimicrob.* **2018**, *17*, 42. [CrossRef]
25. Vollmerhausen, T.L.; Woods, J.L.; Faoagali, J.; Katouli, M. Interactions of uroseptic Escherichia coli with renal (A-498) and gastrointestinal (HT-29) cell lines. *J. Med. Microbiol.* **2014**, *63*, 1575–1583. [CrossRef] [PubMed]
26. Magiorakos, A.; Srinivasan, A.; Carey, R.B.; Carmeli, Y.; Falagas, M.E.; Giske, C.G.; Harbarth, S.; Hindler, J.F. Bacteria: An International Expert Proposal for Interim Standard Definitions for Acquired Resistance. *Microbiology* **2011**, *18*, 268–281. [CrossRef]
27. Patra, N.; Prakash, M.R.; Patil, S.; Rao, M.R. First Case Report of Surgical Site Infection Due to Buttiauxella agrestis in a Neurocare Center in India. *Arch. Med. Health Sci.* **2018**, *6*, 117–119. [CrossRef]
28. Antonello, V.S.; Dallé, J.; Domingues, G.C.; Ferreira, J.A.S.; Fontoura, M.d.C.Q.; Knapp, F.B. Post-cesarean surgical site infection due to Buttiauxella agrestis. *Int. J. Infect. Dis.* **2014**, *22*, 65–66. [CrossRef] [PubMed]
29. Cardentey-Reyes, A.; Jacobs, F.; Struelens, M.J.; Rodriguez-Villalobos, H. First case of bacteremia caused by moellerella wisconsensis: Case report and a review of the literature. *Infection* **2009**, *37*, 544–546. [CrossRef] [PubMed]
30. Shah, B.R.; Hux, J.E. Quantifying the risk of infectious diseases for people with diabetes. *Diabetes Care* **2003**. [CrossRef] [PubMed]
31. Muller, L.M.A.J.; Gorter, K.J.; Hak, E.; Goudzwaard, W.L.; Schellevis, F.G.; Hoepelman, A.I.M.; Rutten, G.E.H.M. Increased Risk of Common Infections in Patients with Type 1 and Type 2 Diabetes Mellitus. *Clin. Infect. Dis.* **2005**, *26*, 510–513. [CrossRef]
32. Lim, J.H.; Cho, J.H.; Lee, J.H.; Park, Y.J.; Jin, S.; Park, G.Y.; Kim, J.S.; Kang, Y.J.; Kwon, O.; Choi, J.Y.; et al. Risk factors for recurrent urinary tract infection in kidney transplant recipients. *Transplant. Pro.* **2013**, *45*, 1584–1589.
33. Rogers, G.B.; Hoffman, L.R.; Whiteley, M.; Daniels, T.W.V.; Carroll, M.P.; Bruce, K.D. Revealing the dynamics of polymicrobial infections: Implications for antibiotic therapy. *Trends Microbiol.* **2010**, *18*, 357–364. [CrossRef]
34. Croxall, G.; Weston, V.; Joseph, S.; Manning, G.; Cheetham, P.; McNally, A. Increased human pathogenic potential of Escherichia coli from polymicrobial urinary tract infections in comparison to isolates from monomicrobial culture samples. *J. Med. Microbiol.* **2011**, *60*, 102–109. [CrossRef]
35. Ranjan, K.P.; Ranjan, N. Citrobacter: An emerging health care associated urinary pathogen. *Urol. Ann.* **2013**, *5*, 313–314. [PubMed]
36. Sami, H.; Sultan, A.; Rizvi, M.; Khan, F.; Ahmad, S.; Shukla, I.; Khan, H. Citrobacter as a uropathogen, its prevalence and antibiotics susceptibility pattern. *CHRISMED J. Heal. Res.* **2017**, *4*, 23. [CrossRef]
37. Aller, A.I.; Castro, C.; Medina, M.J.; González, M.T.; Sevilla, P.; Morilla, M.D.; Corzo, J.E.; Martín-Mazuelos, E. Isolation of Moellerella wisconsensis from blood culture from a patient with acute cholecystitis. *Clin. Microbiol. Infect.* **2009**, *15*, 1193–1194. [CrossRef] [PubMed]
38. Peter, S.; Bezdan, D.; Oberhettinger, P.; Vogel, W.; Dörfel, D.; Dick, J.; Marschal, M.; Liese, J.; Weidenmaier, C.; Autenrieth, I.; et al. Whole-genome sequencing enabling the detection of a colistin-resistant hypermutating Citrobacter werkmanii strain harbouring a novel metallo-β-lactamase VIM-48. *Int. J. Antimicrob. Agents* **2018**, *51*, 867–874. [CrossRef]
39. Duman, M.; Saticioglu, I.B.; Buyukekiz, A.G.; Balta, F.; Altun, S. Molecular characterization and antimicrobial resistance profile of atypical Citrobacter gillenii and Citrobacter sp. isolated from diseased rainbow trout (Oncorhynchus mykiss). *J. Glob. Antimicrob. Resist.* **2017**, *10*, 136–142. [CrossRef]
40. Robino, L.; Scavone, P.; Araujo, L.; Algorta, G.; Zunino, P.; Vignoli, R. Detection of intracellular bacterial communities in a child with Escherichia coli recurrent urinary tract infections. *Pathog. Dis.* **2013**, *68*, 78–81. [CrossRef]
41. Ramírez-Castillo, F.Y.; Moreno-Flores, A.C.; Avelar-González, F.J.; Márquez-Díaz, F.; Harel, J.; Guerrero-Barrera, A.L. An evaluation of multidrug-resistant Escherichia coli isolates in urinary tract infections from Aguascalientes, Mexico: Cross-sectional study. *Ann. Clin. Microbiol. Antimicrob.* **2018**, *17*, 34. [CrossRef]
42. Paniagua-Contreras, G.L.; Monroy-Pérez, E.; Díaz-Velásquez, C.E.; Uribe-García, A.; Labastida, A.; Peñaloza-Figueroa, F.; Domínguez-Trejo, P.; García, L.R.; Vaca-Paniagua, F.; Vaca, S. Whole-genome sequence analysis of multidrug-resistant uropathogenic strains of Escherichia coli from Mexico. *Infect. Drug Resist.* **2019**, *12*, 2363–2377. [CrossRef]
43. Chávez-Jacobo, V.; Ramírez-Díaz, M.; Silva-Sánchez, J.; Cervantes, C. Resistencia Bacteriana a Quinolonas: Determinantes Codificados en Plásmidos. *REB. Rev. Educ. bioquímica* **2015**.
44. Guajardo-Lara, C.E.; González-Martínez, P.M.; Ayala-Gaytán, J.J. Resistencia antimicrobiana en la infección urinaria por Escherichia coli adquirida en la comunidad: ¿Cuál antibiótico voy a usar? *Salud Publica Mex.* **2009**, *51*, 157–161. [CrossRef]
45. Garza-González, E.; Bocanegra-Ibarias, P.; Bobadilla-del-Valle, M.; Ponce-de-León-Garduño, L.A.; Esteban-Kenel, V.; Silva-Sánchez, J.; Garza-Ramos, U.; Barrios-Camacho, H.; López-Jácome, L.E.; Colin-Castro, C.A.; et al. Drug resistance phenotypes and genotypes in Mexico in representative gram-negative species: Results from the infivar network. *PLoS One* **2021**, *16*, e0248614. [CrossRef] [PubMed]

46. Matta-Chuquisapon, J.; Valencia-Bazalar, E.; Marocho-Chahuayo, L.; Gonzales-Escalante, E.; Sevilla-Andrade, C.R. Presencia de genes fimH y afa en aislamientos urinarios de Escherichia coli productora de betalactamasas de espectro extendido en Lima, Perú. *Rev. Peru. Med. Exp. Salud Publica* **2020**, *37*, 282–286. [CrossRef] [PubMed]
47. Dadi, B.R.; Abebe, T.; Zhang, L.; Mihret, A.; Abebe, W.; Amogne, W. Distribution of virulence genes and phylogenetics of uropathogenic Escherichia coli among urinary tract infection patients in Addis Ababa, Ethiopia. *BMC Infect. Dis.* **2020**, *20*, 1–12. [CrossRef]
48. Morales-Espinosa, R.; Hernandez-Castro, R.; Delgado, G.; Mendez, J.L.; Navarro, A.; Manjarrez, A.; Cravioto, A. UPEC strain characterization isolated from Mexican patients with recurrent urinary infections. *J. Infect. Dev. Ctries.* **2016**, *10*, 317–328. [CrossRef]
49. López-Banda, D.A.; Carrillo-Casas, E.M.; Leyva-Leyva, M.; Orozco-Hoyuela, G.; Manjarrez-Hernández, Á.H.; Arroyo-Escalante, S.; Moncada-Barrón, D.; Villanueva-Recillas, S.; Xicohtencatl-Cortes, J.; Hernández-Castro, R. Identification of Virulence Factors Genes in Escherichia coli Isolates from Women with Urinary Tract Infection in Mexico. *Biomed Res. Int.* **2014**, *2014*, 1–10. [CrossRef]
50. Tabasi, M. Genotypic Characterization of Virulence Factors in Escherichia coli Isolated from Patients with Acute Cystitis, Pyelonephritis and Asymptomatic Bacteriuria. *J. Clin. DIAGNOSTIC Res.* **2016**, *12*, DC01–DC07. [CrossRef]
51. Gao, Q.; Zhang, D.; Ye, Z.; Zhu, X.; Yang, W.; Dong, L.; Gao, S.; Liu, X. Virulence traits and pathogenicity of uropathogenic Escherichia coli isolates with common and uncommon O serotypes. *Microb. Pathog.* **2017**, *104*, 217–224. [CrossRef] [PubMed]
52. Ordaz-López, V.I.; Manzo-Banales, H.M.; García-Herrera, H.; Cerda-Rivera, P.E.; Ochoa, M.C.; Ramírez-Leyva, D.H. Urinary Tract Infection in Pregnancy: A Study of Pathogen and Bacterial Resistance in Mexico. *J. Fam. Med.* **2016**, *3*, 1–4.
53. Bravata-Alcantara, J.C.; Bello-Lopez, J.M.; Cortes-Ortiz, I.A.; Mendez-Velazquez, J.J.; Aviles-Soto, B.; Quintas-Granados, L.I.; Chavez-Ocana, S.d.C.; Rosel-Pech, C.; Gonzalez-Barrios, J.A.; Sierra Martinez, M. Distribution of Virulence and Antimicrobial Resistance Genes in Phylogenetic Groups of Escherichia coli Strains Isolated from Mexican Patients with Urinary Infection. *Jundishapur J. Microbiol.* **2019**, In Press. [CrossRef]
54. Luna-Pineda, V.M.; Ochoa, S.A.; Cruz-Córdova, A.; Cázares-Domínguez, V.; Reyes-Grajeda, J.P.; Flores-Oropeza, M.A.; Arellano-Galindo, J.; Castro-Hernández, R.; Flores-Encarnación, M.; Ramírez-Vargas, A.; et al. Features of urinary Escherichia coli isolated from children with complicated and uncomplicated urinary tract infections in Mexico. *PLoS One* **2018**, *13*, e0204934. [CrossRef]
55. Asadi, S.; Kargar, M.; Solhjoo, K.; Najafi, A.; Ghorbani-Dalini, S. The association of virulence determinants of uropathogenic Escherichia coli with antibiotic resistance. *Jundishapur J. Microbiol.* **2014**, *7*, 1–6. [CrossRef]
56. Yun, K.W.; Kim, H.Y.; Park, H.K.; Kim, W.; Lim, I.S. Virulence factors of uropathogenic Escherichia coli of urinary tract infections and asymptomatic bacteriuria in children. *J. Microbiol. Immunol. Infect.* **2014**, *47*, 455–461. [CrossRef]
57. Hernández-Chiñas, U.; Pérez-Ramos, A.; Belmont-Monroy, L.; Chávez-Berrocal, M.E.; González-Villalobos, E.; Navarro-Ocaña, A.; Eslava, C.A.; Molina-Lopez, J. Characterization of auto-agglutinating and non-typeable uropathogenic Escherichia coli strains. *J. Infect. Dev. Ctries.* **2019**, *13*, 465–472. [CrossRef]
58. Dobrindt, U.; Blum-Oehler, G.; Nagy, G.; Schneider, G.; Johann, A.; Gottschalk, G.; Hacker, J. Genetic Structure and Distribution of Four Pathogenicity Islands (PAI I536 to PAI IV536) of Uropathogenic Escherichia coli Strain 536. *Infect. Immun.* **2002**, *70*, 6365–6372. [CrossRef]
59. Manjarrez-Hernandez, A.; Molina-López, J.; Gavilanes-Parra, S.; Hernandez-Castro, R. Escherichia coli clonal group A among uropathogenic infections in Mexico City. *J. Med. Microbiol.* **2016**, *65*, 1438–1444. [CrossRef]
60. Bien, J.; Sokolova, O.; Bozko, P. Role of Uropathogenic Escherichia coli Virulence Factors in Development of Urinary Tract Infection and Kidney Damage. *Int. J. Nephrol.* **2012**, *2012*, 1–15. [CrossRef] [PubMed]
61. Guyer, D.M.; Radulovic, S.; Jones, F.-E.; Mobley, H.L.T. Sat, the Secreted Autotransporter Toxin of Uropathogenic Escherichia coli, Is a Vacuolating Cytotoxin for Bladder and Kidney Epithelial Cells. *Infect. Immun.* **2002**, *70*, 4539–4546. [CrossRef] [PubMed]
62. Frey, J. The role of RTX toxins in host specificity of animal pathogenic Pasteurellaceae. *Vet. Microbiol.* **2011**, *153*, 51–58. [CrossRef]
63. Gur, C.; Coppenhagen-Glazer, S.; Rosenberg, S.; Yamin, R.; Enk, J.; Glasner, A.; Bar-On, Y.; Fleissig, O.; Naor, R.; Abed, J.; et al. Natural killer cell-mediated host defense against uropathogenic E. coli is counteracted by bacterial hemolysinA-dependent killing of NK cells. *Cell Host. Microbe.* **2013**, *14*, 664–674. [CrossRef]
64. Diabate, M.; Munro, P.; Garcia, E.; Jacquel, A.; Michel, G.; Obba, S.; Goncalves, D.; Luci, C.; Marchetti, S.; Demon, D.; et al. Escherichia coli α-Hemolysin Counteracts the Anti-Virulence Innate Immune Response Triggered by the Rho GTPase Activating Toxin CNF1 during Bacteremia. *PLOS Pathog.* **2015**, *11*, e1004732. [CrossRef]

Phenotypic and Molecular Characterization of Commensal, Community-Acquired and Nosocomial *Klebsiella* spp.

Marta Gómez [1], Arancha Valverde [2], Rosa del Campo [2], Juan Miguel Rodríguez [1] and Antonio Maldonado-Barragán [1,3,*]

1. Department of Nutrition and Food Science, Complutense University of Madrid, 28040 Madrid, Spain; marta_gmz@hotmail.com (M.G.); jmrodrig@ucm.es (J.M.R.)
2. Department of Microbiology, Hospital Universitario Ramón y Cajal IRYCIS, 28034 Madrid, Spain; aranchavalverde@gmail.com (A.V.); rosa.campo@salud.madrid.org (R.d.C.)
3. Infection and Global Health Research Division, School of Medicine, University of St. Andrews, North Haugh, St Andrews KY16 9TF, UK
* Correspondence: amb52@st-andrews.ac.uk

Abstract: *Klebsiella* spp. is a relevant pathogen that can present acquired resistance to almost all available antibiotics, thus representing a serious threat for public health. While most studies have been focused on isolates causing community-acquired and nosocomial infections, little is known about the commensal isolates colonizing healthy subjects. We describe the molecular identification and the phenotypic characterization of commensal *Klebsiella* spp. from breast milk of healthy women and faeces from healthy breast-fed infants, which were compared with isolates from community-acquired infections and from a nosocomial NICU outbreak. The phylogenetic analysis of a 454-bp sequence of the *rpoB* gene was useful for species identification (*K. pneumoniae*, *K. variicola*, *K. quasipneumoniae*, *K. oxytoca*, *K. grimontii*, *K. michiganensis*, *Raoultella planticola* and *R. ornithinolytica*), previously misidentified as *K. pneumoniae* or *K. oxytoca* by biochemical methods. Globally, we report that commensal strains present virulence traits (virulence genes, siderophores and biofilms) comparable to community-acquired and NICU-infective isolates, thus suggesting that the human microbiota could constitute a reservoir for infection. Isolates causing NICU outbreak were multi-drug resistant (MDR) and ESBLs producers, although an imipenem-resistant commensal MDR *K. quasipneumoniae* isolate was also found. A commensal *K. pneumoniae* strain showed a potent bacteriocin-like inhibitory activity against MDR *Klebsiella* isolates, thus highlighting the potential role of commensal *Klebsiella* spp. in health and disease.

Keywords: *Klebsiella*; *rpoB*; virulence; siderophores; biofilms; antibiotic resistance; bacteriocins

1. Introduction

Klebsiella spp. are ubiquitous in nature and can be found in environment samples (surface water, sewage, soil and plants) and, also, colonizing the mucosal surfaces of healthy mammals [1]. The major species of this genus is *Klebsiella pneumoniae*, followed by *Klebsiella oxytoca*, both considered as opportunistic pathogens with major relevance in community- and hospital-acquired (nosocomial) infections, which are particularly severe in immunocompromised subjects such as those hospitalized in transplant, intensive care (ICU), or neonatal units (NICU) [2].

Phylogenetic analyses have shown that *K. pneumoniae* complex comprises seven phylogenetic groups (Kp1 to Kp7). Kp1 is the most abundant and includes *K. pneumoniae* sensu stricto; Kp2, Kp3, Kp4, Kp5, Kp6 and Kp7 include *K. quasipneumoniae* subsp. *quasipneumoniae*, *K. variicola* subsp. *variicola*, *K. quasipneumoniae* subsp. *similipneumoniae*, *K. variicola* subsp. *tropicalensis*, *K. quasivariicola* and *K. africanensis*, respectively [3–5]. On the other hand, the *K. oxytoca* complex comprises six phylogroups, Ko1, Ko2, Ko3, Ko4, Ko6 and Ko8, including *K. michiganensis*, *K. oxytoca sensu stricto*, *K. spallanzanii*, *K. pasteurii*, *K. grimonti* and *K. huaxiensis* [4,6].

Isolates grouped in the *K. pneumonie* complex possess similar biochemical and phenotypic features, being inaccurately identified as *K. pneumoniae sensu stricto* or as *K. variicola* by conventional microbiological methods. Thus, a recent study has shown that *K. variicola* and *K. quasipneumoniae*, which are often misidentified as *K. pneumoniae*, cause severe life-threatening infections similar to *K. pneumoniae* [7]. In the same manner, the members of the *K. oxytoca* complex are frequently misidentified as *K. oxytoca sensu stricto*. However, it has been suggested that *K. michiganensis*, which is commonly erroneously identified as *K. oxytoca*, is likely to be more clinically relevant than *K. oxytoca* in human-associated infections [8].

Commensal colonizing isolates have been far less studied than clinically relevant community-acquired and nosocomial *Klebsiella* spp. causing infectious diseases. In fact, studies about commensal *Klebsiella* isolates from healthy non-hospitalized subjects are currently very scarce. By using culture-independent methods, it has been estimated that approximately 3.8% of stool samples from healthy individuals contains *K. pneumoniae* [9]. In a recent study with healthy adults, it has been shown that although *Klebsiella* spp. constitute minor bacterial components of the human gut microbiota, some *K. pneumoniae* isolates could present a great potential to cause infections [10]. This was previously observed in a study with healthy Korean adults, where a high proportion of subjects showed faecal carriage of *K. pneumoniae* sequence type 23, which is associated with pyogenic liver abscess in Korea [11]. In fact, two recent studies with hospitalized adults have shown that gastrointestinal colonization with *K. pneumoniae* is strongly linked to subsequent infections in these subjects during hospitalization and demonstrated that a large proportion of *K. pneumoniae* infections were acquired from patient's own microbiota [12,13].

Nosocomial *Klebsiella* infections are especially problematic in preterm neonates causing neonatal sepsis, including both early- and late-onset infections [14]. In a recent work, it has been shown that "healthy" antibiotic-treated preterm infants hospitalized in NICUs can harbour different *Klebsiella* spp. such as *K. pneumoniae*, *K. quasipneumoniae*, *K. grimontii* and *K. michiganensis*, which could greatly contribute to the resistome [8].

Overall, all these studies suggest that *Klebsiella* spp. is a habitual commensal in the healthy human microbiota, which could provide a potential reservoir for infection. In the light of these findings, the phenotypic and molecular characterization of *Klebsiella* isolates from healthy subjects could contribute to understanding the relevance of commensal *Klebsiella* spp. as a reservoir of potentially dangerous traits for human health. Previous works have determined that this genus can be a part of the human milk microbiota of healthy women [15], frequently arising from the use of pumps for milk expression [16]. Breastfeeding women are a representative sample of the general population since the majority of them will give birth at some point in a hospital, where the newborn will be ideally breastfeed within the first hour of birth. As a consequence, human milk represents one of the first vehicles for the mother-to-infant transfer of microbes [17].

In these studies, we obtained a collection of *Klebsiella* isolates from the milk of healthy women and from the meconium and faeces of breast-fed term infants. The aim of this study was to identify and characterize these commensal *Klebsiella* isolates and compare them with nosocomial isolates from an NICU outbreak and from community-acquired infections isolates.

2. Materials and Methods

2.1. Bacterial Strains and Growth Conditions

A total of 56 *Klebsiella* spp. isolates, which were initially identified as *K. pneumoniae* ($n = 35$) or *K. oxytoca* ($n = 21$) by routine biochemical methods (Wider system; Francisco Soria Melguizo, S.A., Madrid, Spain), were included in this study (Table 1). These isolates were obtained from different origins: (i) 20 commensal isolates from human milk ($n = 5$), meconium ($n = 1$) and faeces of breast-fed infants ($n = 14$) of healthy individuals from the bacterial collection of the research group 920080 (Complutense University of Madrid, Spain); (ii) 26 community-acquired isolates causing bacteraemia in adult outpatients at the Hospital Ramón y Cajal (Madrid, Spain); and (iii) 10 clinical isolates from the neonatal ICU of the Hospital 12 de Octubre (Madrid, Spain) from blood (n = 2), catheter (n = 1), environmental surfaces (n = 2) and colonizing the gut of newborns admitted at NICU (n = 5). The Ethical Committee on Clinical Research of the Hospital Clínico San Carlos of Madrid (Spain) approved the study protocol (reference 10/017-E). In the frame of such protocol, samples used to isolate the bacterial strains were obtained after informed written consent of each person or, when required, of the infants' legal guardians. All strains were routinely grown in Brain Heart Infusion (BHI; Oxoid, Basingstoke, UK) broth, BHI solid medium (containing 1.5% w/v agar) and MacConkey agar medium (BioMèrieux, Marcy l'Etoile, Francia) at 37 °C for 24 h. *K. pneumoniae* subsp. *pneumoniae* DSMZ30104^T, *K. pneumoniae* subsp. *rhinoscleromatis* DSMZ16231^T, *K. pneumoniae* subsp. *ozaenae* DSMZ16358^T, *K. pneumoniae* CECT 142, *K. pneumoniae* CECT 517 and *K. oxytoca* CECT 860^T were used as reference strains.

Table 1. Biochemical and molecular identification (based on partial *rpoB* gene sequencing) of commensal, community-acquired, NICU outbreak and reference strains used in this study.

Strains	Biochemical ID	*rpoB* (% Identity)	Origin	Source *
Commensal				
HA001	*K. oxytoca*	*K. michiganensis* (100)	Faeces	UCM
HA009	*K. oxytoca*	*K. michiganensis* (100)	Faeces	UCM
HI2-45	*K. oxytoca*	*K. michiganensis* (100)	Faeces	UCM
HV1-02	*K. oxytoca*	*K. michiganensis* (99.52)	Faeces	UCM
HV1-11	*K. oxytoca*	*K. michiganensis* (99.52)	Faeces	UCM
HV2-03	*K. oxytoca*	*K. michiganensis* (99.52)	Faeces	UCM
HV2-11	*K. oxytoca*	*K. michiganensis* (99.52)	Faeces	UCM
LG5-52	*K. oxytoca*	*K. michiganensis* (99.52)	Milk	UCM
MV11	*K. oxytoca*	*K. michiganensis* (99.52)	Meconium	UCM
LMV2-9	*K. pneumoniae*	*K. pneumoniae* (99.76)	Milk	UCM
LMV6-5	*K. pneumoniae*	*K. pneumoniae* (99.76)	Milk	UCM
LMV90-10	*K. pneumoniae*	*K. pneumoniae* (100)	Milk	UCM
LMV90-11	*K. pneumoniae*	*K. pneumoniae* (100)	Milk	UCM
MV3-1	*K. pneumoniae*	*K. variicola* (100)	Faeces	UCM
MV31-21	*K. pneumoniae*	*K. pneumoniae* (99.76)	Faeces	UCM
MV91-1	*K. pneumoniae*	*K. pneumoniae* (99.76)	Faeces	UCM
MV91-24	*K. pneumoniae*	*K. quasipneumoniae* subsp. *similipneumoniae* (100)	Faeces	UCM
MV91-25	*K. pneumoniae*	*K. pneumoniae* (99.76)	Faeces	UCM
MV91-28	*K. pneumoniae*	*K. pneumoniae* (100)	Faeces	UCM
MV91-42	*K. pneumoniae*	*K. quasipneumoniae* subsp. *quasipneumoniae* (99.52)	Faeces	UCM
Community-acquired				
Ko1	*K. pneumoniae*	*R. planticola* (100)	Blood culture	RYC
Ko2	*K. oxytoca*	*K. michiganensis* (99.76)	Blood culture	RYC
Ko3	*K. oxytoca*	*K. michiganensis* (99.52)	Blood culture	RYC
Ko4	*K. oxytoca*	*K. michiganensis* (100)	Blood culture	RYC
Ko5	*K. oxytoca*	*K. michiganensis* (100)	Blood culture	RYC
Ko6	*K. oxytoca*	*K. michiganensis* (99.76)	Blood culture	RYC
Ko7	*K. oxytoca*	*K. oxytoca* (100)	Blood culture	RYC
Ko8	*K. oxytoca*	*K. grimontii* (98.80)	Blood culture	RYC
Ko9	*K. oxytoca*	*K. pneumoniae* (99.76)	Blood culture	RYC
Ko10	*K. oxytoca*	*R. ornithinolytica* (100)	Blood culture	RYC
Ko11	*K. oxytoca*	*K. grimontii* (99.04)	Blood culture	RYC
Ko12	*K. oxytoca*	*K. michiganensis* (99.52)	Blood culture	RYC
Kp1	*K. pneumoniae*	*K. pneumoniae* (99.76)	Blood culture	RYC

Table 1. Cont.

Strains	Biochemical ID	rpoB (% Identity)	Origin	Source *
Kp2	K. pneumoniae	K. pneumoniae (99.52)	Blood culture	RYC
Kp3	K. pneumoniae	K. pneumoniae (99.76)	Blood culture	RYC
Kp4	K. pneumoniae	K. pneumoniae (99.76)	Blood culture	RYC
Kp5	K. pneumoniae	K. pneumoniae (99.76)	Blood culture	RYC
Kp6	K. pneumoniae	K. pneumoniae (100)	Blood culture	RYC
Kp7	K. pneumoniae	K. pneumoniae (99.76)	Blood culture	RYC
Kp8	K. pneumoniae	K. pneumoniae (100)	Blood culture	RYC
Kp9	K. pneumoniae	K. pneumoniae (99.76)	Blood culture	RYC
Kp10	K. pneumoniae	K. pneumoniae (99.76)	Blood culture	RYC
Kp12	K. pneumoniae	K. pneumoniae (99.76)	Blood culture	RYC
Kp13	K. pneumoniae	K. pneumoniae (99.76)	Blood culture	RYC
Kp14	K. pneumoniae	K. pneumoniae (99.76)	Blood culture	RYC
Kp15	K. pneumoniae	K. pneumoniae (100)	Blood culture	RYC
NICU outbreak				
K12-1	K. pneumoniae	K. pneumoniae (100)	Blood culture	HUDO
K12-2	K. pneumoniae	K. pneumoniae (100)	Blood culture	HUDO
K12-3	K. pneumoniae	K. variicola (99.52)	NICU environment	HUDO
K12-4	K. pneumoniae	K. pneumoniae (99.76)	NICU environment	HUDO
K12-5	K. pneumoniae	K. michiganensis (100)	Faeces	HUDO
K12-6	K. pneumoniae	K. pneumoniae (100)	Vascular catheter	HUDO
K12-7	K. oxytoca	K. michiganensis (100)	Faeces	HUDO
K12-8	K. pneumoniae	K. pneumoniae (99.76)	Faeces	HUDO
K12-9	K. pneumoniae	K. pneumoniae (99.76)	Faeces	HUDO
K12-10	K. pneumoniae	K. pneumoniae (99.76)	Faeces	HUDO
Reference type strains ([T])				
DSM 30104[T]	K. pneumoniae subsp. pneumoniae	K. pneumoniae (100)	Unknown	DSMZ
CECT 142	K. pneumoniae subsp. pneumoniae	K. pneumoniae (99.76)	Unknown	CECT
CECT 517	K. pneumoniae subsp. pneumoniae	K. pneumoniae (100)	Urine	CECT
DSM 16231[T]	K. pneumoniae subsp. rhinoscleromatis	K. pneumoniae (100)	Nose rhinoscleroma	DSMZ
DSM 16358[T]	K. pneumoniae subsp. ozaenae	K. pneumoniae (100)	Nose	DSMZ
CECT 860[T]	K. oxytoca	K. oxytoca (100)	Pharyngeal tonsil	CECT

Abbreviations: * UCM, group 920080, Complutense University of Madrid; RYC, Hospital Universitario Ramón y Cajal; HUDO, Hospital Universitario 12 de Octubre; CECT, Spanish Type Culture Collection; DSMZ, German Collection of Microorganisms and Cell Cultures GmbH.

2.2. Molecular Identification of Isolates

All isolates were re-identified by sequencing a 454-bp fragment of the *rpoB* gene amplified by PCR with KrpoB-for and KrpoB-rev primer pair (Table S1). PCR conditions were as follows: 1 cycle of 94 °C for 4 min, 30 cycles of 94 °C for 30 s, 55 °C for 30 s and 72 °C for 30 s and a final extension of 72 °C for 5 min. Amplicons were purified using the Nucleospin Extract II kit (Macherey-Nagel, Düren, Germany) and sequenced (ABI Prism 3730; Applied Biosystems, Foster City, CA, USA) at the Genomics Unit of the Universidad Complutense de Madrid (Madrid, Spain). The resulting sequences were used to search against reference sequences deposited in the EMBL database using BLASTn algorithm (http://www.ncbi.nlm.nih.gov; accessed on 7 July 2021). The identity of the isolates was determined on the basis of the highest scores. The *rpoB* gene sequences obtained were deposited in the GenBank database, under the accession numbers KJ499842 to KJ499903.

2.3. Phylogenetic Analysis

For phylogenetic analysis, the *rpoB* sequences obtained were aligned by using the Clustal W method [18] with the MEGA version 6 (Revision 6.06, update February 2014) software created by Tamura, Stecher, Peterson, Filipski, and Kumar [19]. Phylogenetic trees were constructed based on the neighbour-joining method with the Jukes–Cantor parameter model [20]. Bootstraping analysis (1000 replicates) was performed to study the stability of the groupings. The *rpoB* sequences of the following type species were obtained from the GenBank database and included in the phylogenetic analysis the following: *K. variicola* F2R9^T (AY367356), *Raoultella ornithinolytica* ATCC 31898^T (AF129447), *Raoultella planticola* ATCC 33531^T (AF129449) and *Staphylococcus sciuri* subsp. *carnaticus* ATCC 700058^T (DQ120748).

2.4. Genotyping of Isolates

Pulsed-field gel electrophoresis (PFGE) was performed as described previously [21]. Chromosomal DNA of each isolate was digested with 30 U of XbaI (TaKaRa Bio Inc, Shiga, Japan). Electrophoresis was carried out in a CHEF DR II apparatus (Bio-Rad, Laboratories, Hercules, CA, USA) with the following conditions: 14 °C, 6 V/cm^2 and 10–40 s for 24 h. Dendrograms of genetic relationships were constructed by using the Phoretix 1D software (version 5.0; Nonlinear Dynamics Ltd., Newcastle upon Tyne, UK) based on the Dice coefficient.

Small plasmids were extracted from 16 h BHI broth cultures with the "QIAprep Spin Miniprep Kit" (QIAgen) as recommended by the manufacturer and visualized in a 1% agarose gel by using conventional electrophoresis (90 V for 90 min). Supercoiled ladder (1–16 kb) (Invitrogen, Paisley, UK) was used as molecular weight marker. Large plasmids (>16 kb) were extracted using PFGE-S1 nuclease digestion (Takara Bio Inc, Shiga, Japan) with the following conditions: 14 °C, 6 V/cm^2 and 5–25 s for 3 h followed by 30–45 s for 12 h. Size was determined using the Lambda Ladder PFG Marker (48.5–1000, 18 Kb) and Low Range PFG Marker (0.13–194 Kb) (New England Biolabs, Inc.) as references. The resulting plasmid profiles were graphically represented and analysed using the software available on http://insilico.ehu.es/dice_upgma/ (accessed on 7 July 2021) to generate dendrograms by UPGMA clustering using Dice correlation.

2.5. Antimicrobial Susceptibility Testing

Minimal inhibitory concentrations (MICs) to antibiotics were evaluated by a microdilution method using the Sensititre EMIZA 9EF (TREK Diagnostic Systems, Cleveland, EEUU) plates following the manufacturer's instructions. Production of Extended-spectrum β-lactamases (ESBLs) was tested by the double-disk synergy test [22] containing ceftazidime/ceftazidime plus clavulanate or cefotaxime/cefotaxime plus clavulanate. The presence of CTX-M β-lactamase-encoding genes (*bla*$_{CTX-M}$) was identified by multiplex PCR using the oligonucleotides CTX-M-1G-F, CTX-M-1G-R, CTX-M-2G-F, CTX-M-2G-R, CTX-M-9G-F and CTX-M-9G-R (Table S1) and conditions described previously [23]. P1 and P2b primers (Table S1) were used to amplify *bla*$_{CTX-M}$ subgroup I genes [24]. Multidrug-resistance (MDR) was defined as non-susceptibility (resistance) to at least one agent in three or more antimicrobial categories [25].

2.6. Virulence Determinants

Presence of the *magA*, *rmpA*, *wabG*, *uge*, *kfu* and *fimH* genes encoding potential virulence factors was determined by PCR using specific primers (Table S1) and conditions described previously [26,27]. A novel multiplex PCR was designed to detect genes associated to biosynthesis or receptors of the siderophores aerobactin (*iutA*, *iucB*), enterobactin (*fepA*, *fepC*) and yersibactin (*fyuA*, *ybtT*). For this purpose, six oligonucleotide pairs were designed (iutA-F/iutA-R, iucB-F/iucB-R, fepA-F/fepA-R, fepC-F/fepC-R, FyuA-F/FyuA-R and YbtT-F/YbtT-R; Table S1), which result in the amplification of DNA fragments of 580, 692, 897, 280, 828 and 451 bp, respectively. PCR conditions were as follows: 1 cycle of 94 °C for 4 min, 30 cycles of 94 °C for 30 s, 62 °C for 30 s, 72 °C for 1 min and a final extension of 72 °C for 5 min.

2.7. Hypermucoviscosity, Biofilms, Siderophores and Bacteriocin Activity Assays

The hypermucoviscous phenotype was determined by the string test [28]. The biofilm formation ability was analysed in polyvinylchloride plastic (PVC) microtiter plates as described previously [29,30]. Siderophores production was quantified in cell-free supernatants [31]. The ability to inhibit the growth of other strains by production of bacteriocin-like substances was tested both on solid and broth medium, according to the direct [32] and the "spot-on-the-lawn" methods [33], respectively.

3. Results

3.1. Molecular Identification of Klebsiella Species

The amplification and sequencing of a 454 bp fragment of the *rpoB* gene achieved a great level of discrimination of the *Klebsiella* isolates at the species level when compared against the *rpoB* sequences from the validated type strains (Table 1). Among the 21 isolates initially identified as *K. oxytoca* by routine biochemical methods, just 1 isolate was identified as *K. oxytoca sensu stricto* by *rpoB* sequencing. The rest of the isolates were identified as *K. michiganensis* (n = 16), *K. grimontii* (n = 2), *K. pneumoniae* (n = 1) and *R. ornithinolytica* (n = 1). In the case of the 35 *Klebsiella* isolates initially identified as *K. pneumoniae* by biochemical methods, most of them were identified as *K. pneumoniae sensu stricto* (n= 29) based on *rpoB* sequencing; the remaining isolates were identified as *K. variicola* (n = 2), *K. quasipneumoniae* subsp. *similipneumoniae* (n = 1), *K. quasipneumoniae* subsp. *quasipneumoniae* (n = 1), *K. michiganensis* (n = 1) and *Raoultella planticola* (n = 1). The reference strains *K. pneumoniae* subsp. *pneumoniae* DSMZ30104^T, *K. pneumoniae* subsp. *rhinoscleromatis* DSMZ16231T, *K. pneumoniae* subsp. *ozaenae* DSMZ16358^T, *K. pneumoniae* CECT 142, *K. pneumoniae* CECT 517 and *K. oxytoca* CECT 860^T were correctly identified to the species level by *rpoB* sequencing.

3.2. Phylogenetic Analysis Based on rpoB

The phylogenetic analysis based on the partial amplification of the rpoB gene, supported the molecular identification of all Klebsiella isolates. Indeed, all *K. pneumoniae* isolates clustered with phylogenetic group KpI (*K. pneumoniae*), while isolates MV91-24 and MV91-42 clustered with KpII-A (*K. quasipneumoniae* subsp. *similipneumoniae*) and KpII-B (*K. quasipneumoniae* subsp. *quasipneumoniae*), respectively. The MV3-1 and K12-3 isolates clustered with KpIII (*K. variicola* subsp. *varicola*). All isolates identified as *K. michiganensis* clustered with phylogroup KoI (*K. michiganensis*), while isolate Ko7 clustered with KoII (*K. oxytoca*) and isolates Ko8 and Ko11 clustered with KoIV (*K. grimontii*). The two identified Raoultella isolates, Ko1 and Ko10, clustered with *R. planticola* and with *R. ornithinolytica*, respectively (Figure 1).

3.3. Genetic Diversity

A high genetic diversity among the *K. pneumoniae* and the *K. oxytoca* complex isolates was detected by PFGE (Figure S1). However, within the *K. pneumoniae* isolates, two clonal groups (>80% similarity) were identified: CP1, formed by *K. pneumoniae* K12-1, K12-6 and K12-8, and CP2, formed by *K. pneumoniae* K12-4 and K12-9 (Figure S1A). All these clonal isolates were isolated from the NICU's outbreak. In the *K. oxytoca* complex, we identified two clonal groups (CM1 and CM2), formed by *K. michiganensis* HA001 and HA009, and *K. michiganensis* HV1-02 and HV2-11, respectively (Figure S1B). Those isolates were isolated from faeces from breast-fed healthy term infants.

Plasmid profiles showed that a total of 28 (89%) isolates from the *K. pneumoniae* complex (Figure S2A) and 18 (85%) from the *K. oxytoca* complex (Figure S2B) contained plasmids (1 to 8 plasmids, ranging from 1 to 600 kb).

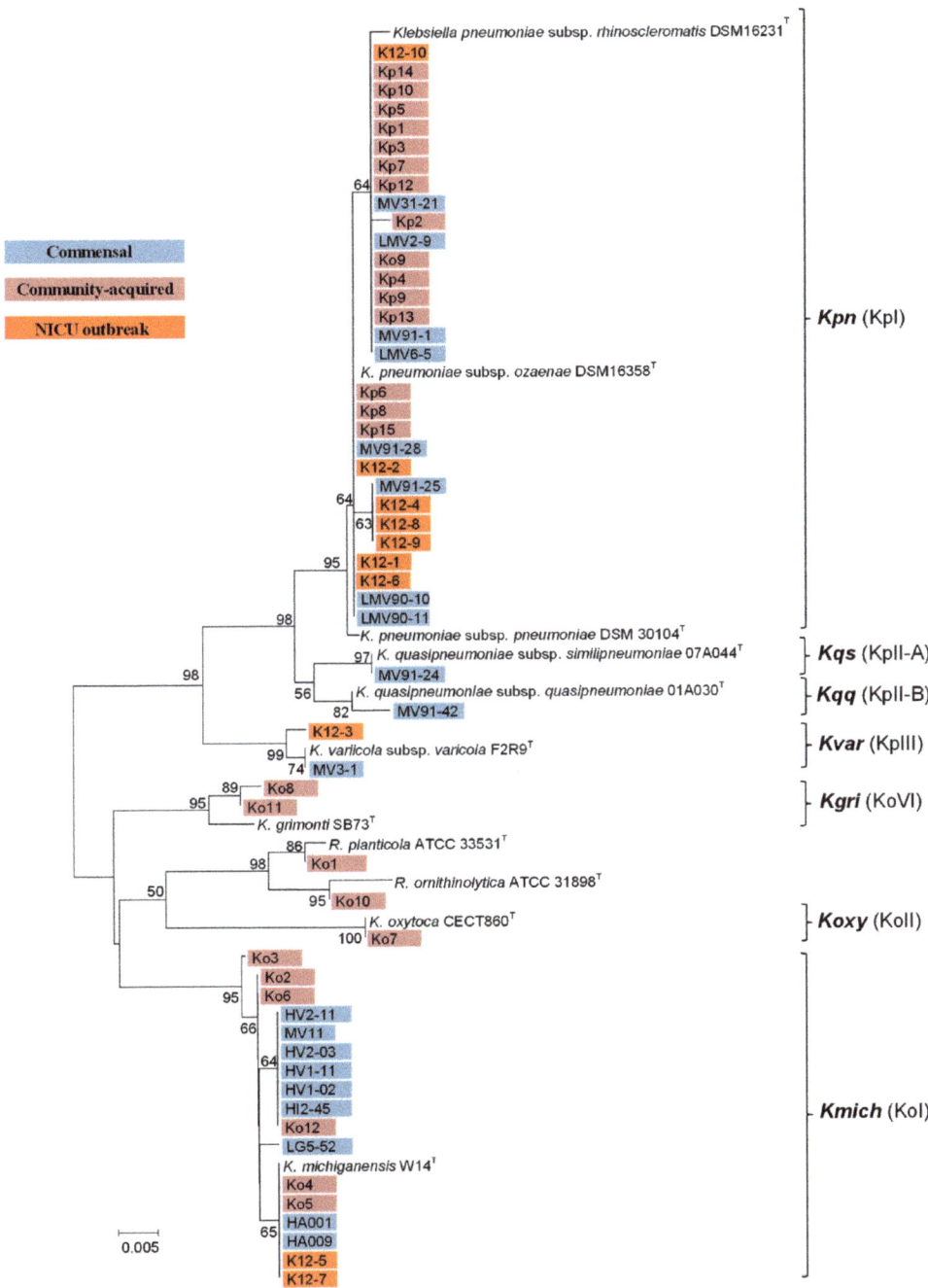

Figure 1. Phylogenetic relationships of 56 *Klebsiella* isolates and reference type strains by comparison of partial *rpoB* gene sequences (454 bp): The tree was based on the neighbour-joining method, using the Jukes–Cantor parameter model. Numbers on the tree indicate bootstrap values calculated for 1000 subsets for branch-points greater than 50%. Bar, 0.005 nucleotide changes per nucleotide position. Phylogenetic groups (KpI, KpII-A, KpII-B, KpIII, KoII, KoVI and KoI) are shown in brackets (Kpn: *K. pneumoniae*; Kqs: *K. quasipneumoniae* subsp. *similipneumoniae*; Kqq: *K. quasipneumoniae* subsp. *quasipneumoniae*; Kvar: *K. variicola*; Kgri: *Klebsiella grimontii*; Koxy: *K. oxytoca*; Kmich: *K. michiganensis*).

3.4. Antimicrobial Susceptibility

Low antibiotic resistance rates were detected in both commensal and bacteraemic community-acquired collections (Figure 2). The isolates were susceptible to most antibiotics tested with the exception of *K. quasipneumoniae* subsp. *similipneumoniae* MV91-24, an MDR and imipenem-resistant isolate from faeces of a healthy breast-fed infant, and *K. pneumoniae* Kp9 and *K. michiganensis* Ko12, two MDR isolates from community-acquired infections.

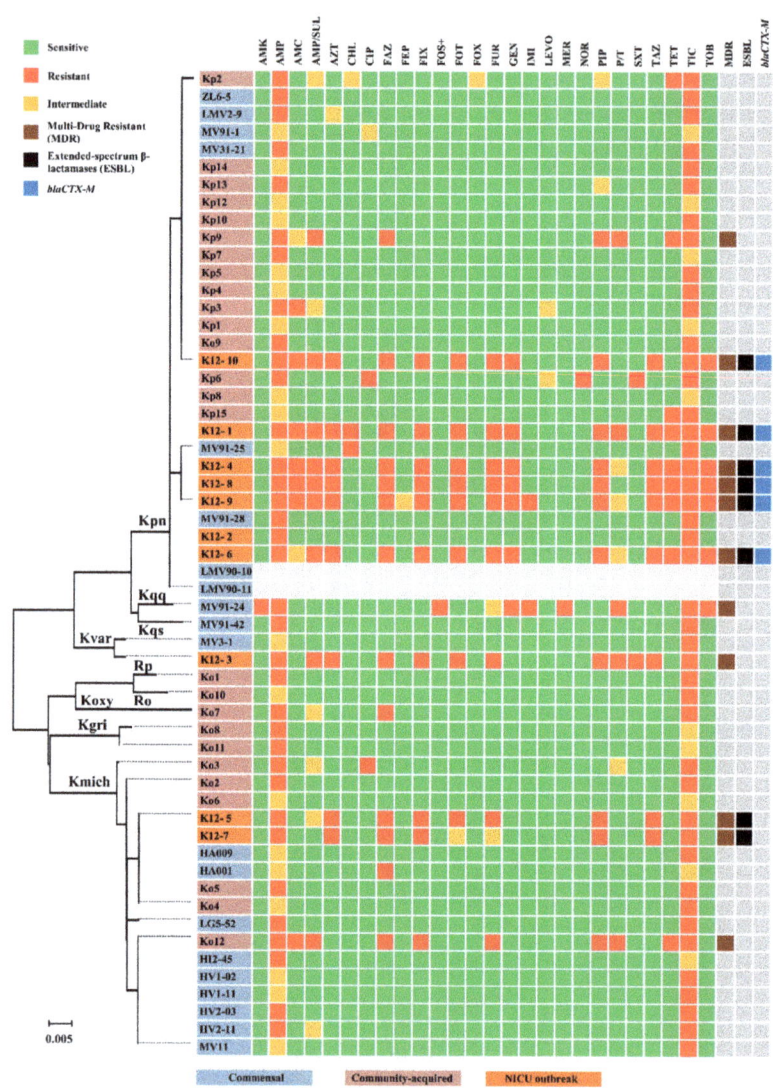

Figure 2. Antibiotic resistance profiles among the Klebsiella isolates analysed in this study: Antibiotics: amikacin (AMK), ampicillin (AMP), amoxicillin–clavulanic acid (AMC), ampicillin-sulbactam (AMP/SUL), aztreonam (AZT), chloramphenicol (CHL), ciprofloxacin (CIP), cefazolin (FAZ), cefepime (FEP), cefixime (FIX), fosfomycin (FOS), cefotaxime (FOT), cefoxitin (FOX), cefuroxime (FUR), gentamicin (GEN), imipenem (IMI), levofloxacin (LEVO), meropenem (MER), norfloxacin (NOR), piperacillin (PIP), piperacillin-tazobactam (P/T), trimethoprim-sulfamethoxazole (SXT), ceftazidime (TAZ), tetracycline (TET), ticarcillin (TIC) and tobramycin (TOB).

All isolates from the NICU showed a MDR phenotype, including ESBL production, with the unique exception of *K. pneumoniae* K12-2 (Figure 2). The antibiotic susceptibility profiles of *K. pneumoniae* K12-1, K12-4, K12-6, K12-8, K12-9 and K12-10, *K. michiganensis* K12-5 and K12-7 and *K. variicola* K12-3 were compatible with ESBLs production, a fact that was subsequently confirmed by the double-disk synergy test and the presence of the $bla_{CTX-M-15}$ gene.

3.5. Virulence Determinants, Hypermucoviscosity, Biofilms and Siderophores

The presence of the wabG, uge and kfu genes was detected in 38.2%, 38.2% and 20.6% of the isolates from the *K. pneumoniae* complex, respectively (Figure 3). The wabG gene was more represented among commensal than among community-acquired isolates ($p < 0.05$), while the uge gene was more abundant among the NICU outbreak isolates than among the community-acquired ones ($p > 0.05$). All members of the *K. pneumoniae* complex presented the fimH gene (with the exception of *K. pneumoniae* Ko9), whereas the magA and rmpA genes were not detected. In contrast, none of the isolates from the *K. oxytoca* complex contained any of the virulence genes studied by PCR.

A novel multiplex PCR targeting the biosynthesis and receptor genes of the siderophores aerobactin, enterobactin and yersibactin (Figure 3) showed that among the *K. pneumoniae* complex, 64.7% presented the fepA gene (enterobactin synthesis), 79.4% the fepC (enterobactin receptor), 14.7% the fyuA (yersibactin synthesis) and 14.7% the ybtT (yersibactin receptor). None of the isolates harboured the genes iutA and iucB encoding the synthesis and receptor genes of aerobactin. The fepC gene was more represented among commensal than among community-acquired isolates ($p < 0.05$).

Within the *K. oxytoca* complex, the fepA gene was not detected in any of the isolates, while the fepC gene was present in 55% of the isolates. The genes fyuA and ybtT were detected in 55% and 5% of the isolates. The fyuA gene was less represented among community-acquired than among commensal isolates ($p < 0.05$). The iucB gene encoding the aerobactin receptor was only detected in two isolates.

None of the Klebsiella isolates showed a hypermucoviscous phenotype. Only 14.7 % of the isolates from the *K. pneumoniae* complex (all belonging to *K. pneumoniae*) were able to grow on biofilms formation on PVC plates (Figure 3), while none of the isolates from the *K. oxytoca* group showed this property. No significant differences were found in the ability to produce siderophores when comparing the isolates from the *K. pneumoniae* and *K. oxytoca* complex. However, commensal isolates produced more siderophores than community-acquired isolates ($p > 0.05$).

3.6. Antimicrobial Activity

Antimicrobial activity was only produced by the commensal *K. pneumoniae* MV91-1 and the community-acquired *K. pneumoniae* Kp5 isolates (Figure 4). MV91-1 showed a wide inhibitory spectrum against the other Klebsiella isolates, being active against *K. pneumoniae*, *K. quasipneumoniae* subsp. *similipneumoniae*, *K. pneumoniae* subsp. *quasipneumoniae*, *K. variicola*, *R. ornithinolytica*, *K. grimontii* and *K. michiganensis* (Figure 3). In contrast, the inhibitory spectrum of Kp5 was narrower, being active only against *K. pneumoniae*, *K. variicola* and *K. michiganensis* (Figure 3). The inhibitory activity of both strains was displayed only on solid medium and was abolished after the addition of proteinase K (1 mg/mL final concentration).

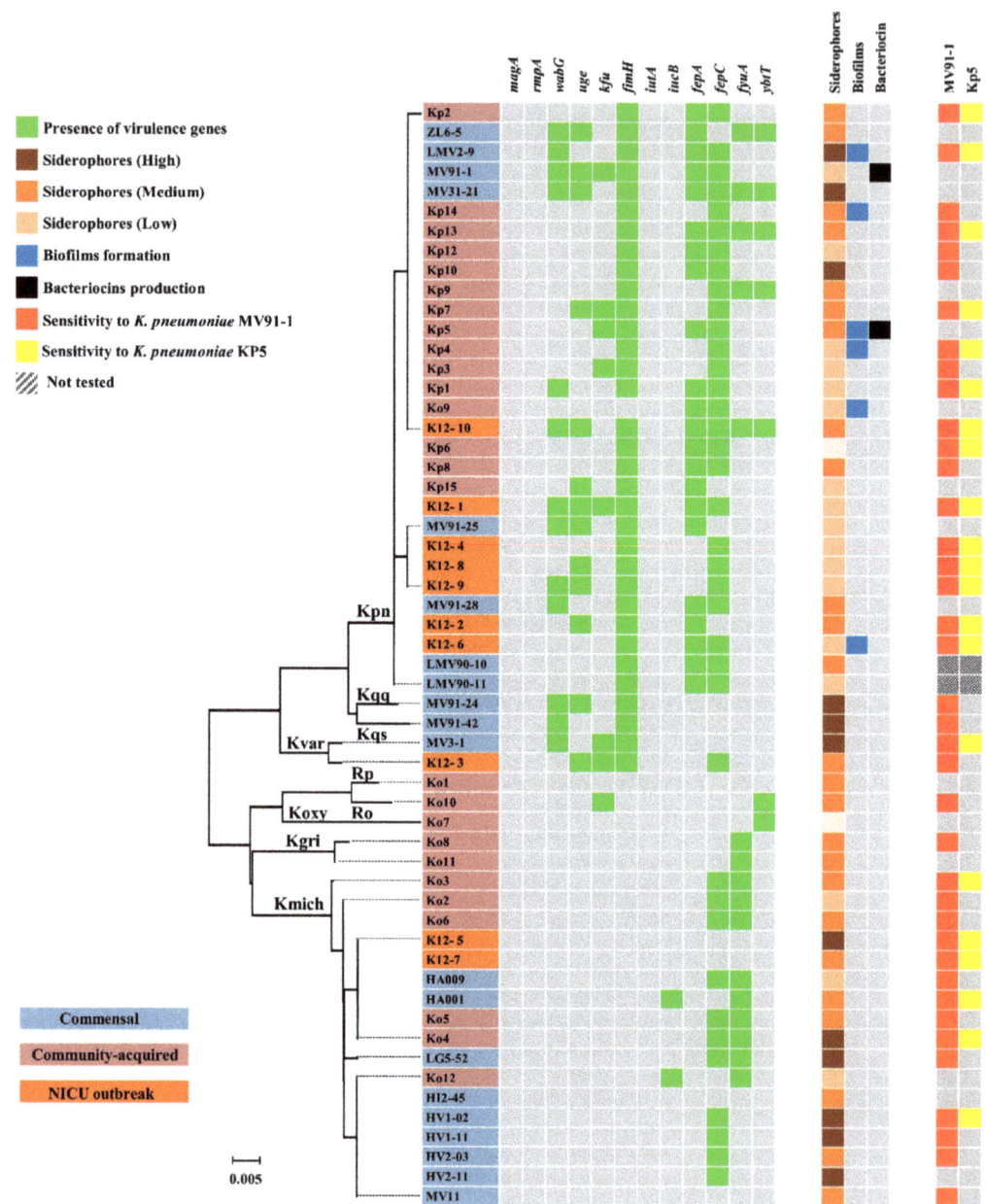

Figure 3. Virulence genes and phenotypic features of the *Klebsiella* isolates analysed in this study: The presence of genes involved in virulence, i.e., *magA* and *rmpA* (hypermucoviscosity phenotype), *wabG* (lipopolysaccharide synthesis), *uge* (uridine diphosphate galacturonate 4-epimerase), *kfu* (iron-uptake system), *fimH* (type 1 fimbrial adhesin), *iutA* (siderophore Aerobactin), *iut B* (receptor of Aerobactin), *fepA* (siderophore Enterobactin), *fepC* (receptor of Enterobactin), *fyuA* (siderophore Yersibactin), *ybtT* (receptor of Yersibactin), was determined by PCR. Production of siderophores was quantified in cell-free supernatants; biofilm formation was assayed and quantified in PVC microtiter plates; production of proteinaceous antimicrobial compounds (bacteriocins) was tested on solid culture medium against all *Klebsiella* isolates of this study, used as indicator strains. Sensitivity to bacteriocins produced by *K. pneumoniae* MV91-1 and Kp5 was assayed on solid medium.

MV91-1 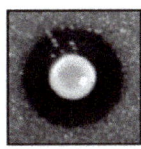   Kp5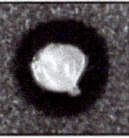

Figure 4. Antimicrobial activity of *K. pneumoniae* MV91-1 (commensal) and Kp5 (community-acquired) against *K. pneumoniae* K12-9, a multidrug ESBL-producer isolate from NICU.

4. Discussion

Species from the genus *Klebsiella*, such as *K. pneumoniae* or *K. oxytoca*, are well-known for their ability to cause a wide range of infections in humans, some of them with fatal consequences [1]. An additional concern is that *Klebsiella* spp. has readily developed antimicrobial resistance to multiple antibiotics, being difficult to treat and eliminate with current antibiotics, thus generating a serious threat to public health [34]. Although most studies have been focused on the study of *Klebsiella* isolates from clinical samples (nosocomial and community-acquired infections), recent studies have shown that our own gastrointestinal tract is a potential reservoir of *Klebsiella* isolates, making difficult the delimitation between pathogens and commensal isolates [10–13]. This, together with the increasing number of novel *Klebsiella* species associated with humans that could cause severe infections, requires the development of new studies focused on the identification and characterization of commensal *Klebsiella* isolates from healthy subjects.

A proper identification of *Klebsiella* isolates at the species level is relevant from an epidemiological and clinical point of view, but routine biochemical tests have limitations since members of this genus possess similar biochemical and phenotypic features. Molecular identification based on ribosomal 16S rDNA gene sequences has been useful in defining bacterial relationships, including those of *Klebsiella* [35]; however, their value for delineating closely related species seems limited because of the scarce nucleotide variation. The identification of *Klebsiella* species and phylogenetic groups within *K. pneumoniae* and *K. oxytoca* based on molecular methods can now be reliably achieved based on the sequencing of housekeeping genes such as *rpoB*, *gyrA* and *parC* [4,5,36].

In this work, we have shown that the amplification and sequencing of a 454 bp fragment of the *rpoB* gene achieved a great level of discrimination for the identification of *Klebsiella* isolates, which was supported by the phylogenetic analysis, thus providing a fast and reliable tool to identify species belonging to this genus. Among the 35 isolates identified as *K. pneumoniae* by biochemical methods, 29 were identified as *K. pneumoniae* sensu stricto based on *rpoB*, while the remaining 6 corresponded to *K. variicola* ($n = 2$), *K. quasipneumoniae* subsp. *similipneumoniae* ($n = 1$), *K. quasipneumoniae* subsp. *quasipneumoniae* ($n = 1$), *K. michiganensis* ($n = 1$) and *R. planticola* ($n = 1$) (Table 1). Although most *K. pneumoniae* were correctly identified by routine biochemical approaches, the misidentification of *K. variicola* and *K. quasipneumoniae* as *K. pneumoniae* is according to the results provided by previous studies [5,7,8,37]. This should be carefully considered since *K. variicola* and *K. quasipneumoniae* can cause severe life-threatening infections similar to *K. pneumoniae* [7,8]. On the other hand, most of the isolates identified by biochemical methods as *K. oxytoca* (16 of 21) were identified as *K. michiganensis* based on *rpoB*, while the remaining 5 were classified as *K. grimontii* ($n = 2$), *K. pneumoniae* ($n = 1$), *K. oxytoca* sensu stricto ($n = 1$) and *R. ornithinolytica* ($n = 1$). Thus, just 1 of the 21 isolates identified as *K. oxytoca* by routine biochemical approaches was *K. oxytoca* sensu stricto, while the vast majority belonged to *K. michiganensis*. These results support the findings of a recent study that have suggested that *K. michiganensis* could be more clinically relevant than *K. oxytoca* in human-associated infections [8]. This misidentification could have hidden the actual clinical and epidemiological significance of these species and, therefore, the implementation of alternative taxonomic methods, such as the sequencing of the *rpoB* gene, should be encouraged in clinical microbiology laboratories.

Interestingly, we found a great variety of commensal *Klebsiella* spp. isolated from healthy subjects (milk from lactating women and faeces from breast-fed infants), such as *K. pneumoniae*, *K. quapsineumoniae* subsp *similipneumoniae* and *K. quapsineumoniae* subsp *quasipneumoniae*, *K. variicola* and *K. michiganensis*. This is in line with a recent study where it has been described that "healthy" antibiotic-treated preterm infants hospitalized in NICUs can harbour different *Klebsiella* species, including *K. pneumoniae*, *K. quasipneumoniae*, *K. grimontii* and *K. michiganensis* [8]. Similarly, *K. pneumoniae* and *K. oxytoca* have been described as components of the human gut microbiota from healthy adults [9–11]. With respect to community-acquired infections, we also found a great variety of species, such as *K. pneumoniae*, *K. oxytoca*, *K. michiganensis*, *K. grimontii*, *R. planticola* and *R. ornithinolytica*. Although *Raoultella* spp. are infrequent human pathogens, *R. ornithinolytica* is considered as emerging bacteria causing human infections [38,39]. The low prevalence of *R. ornithinolytica*- and *R. planticola*-related infections could be due to their misidentification as *K. pneumoniae* or *K. oxytoca* by conventional biochemical tests. In relation to the isolates from the NICU outbreak, we found two *K. michiganensis* strains (K12-5 and K12-7) that had been misidentified as *K. pneumoniae* and *K. oxytoca*, respectively. A recent study reported, for the first time, an NICU nosocomial outbreak caused by MDR and ESBL-producing *K. michiganensis* isolates [40]. This could indicate that hospital outbreaks caused by *K. michiganensis* could have passed undetected due their misclassification as other *Klebsiella* species. In addition, we found that an NICU's isolate (K12-3) previously misidentified as *K. pneumoniae* actually belonged to *K. variicola*, which is currently considered as an emerging human pathogen [7,41]

A high genetic diversity was found among the commensal and the community-acquired *Klebsiella* isolates, whereas those from the NICU seemed to be the result of a polyclonal dissemination. Globally, the commensal and community-acquired *Klebsiella* isolates were sensitive to most of the antibiotics assayed in this study, with the exception of the commensal MV91-24 (*K. quasipneumoniae* subsp. *similipneumoniae*), and the community-acquired Ko12 (*K. michiganensis*) and Kp9 (*K. pneumoniae*), which were multi-drug-resistant (MDR). In contrast, 9 out of the 10 *Klebsiella* isolates from the NICU were MDR, thus supporting the situation of nosocomial outbreak. In addition, the NICU $bla_{CTX-M-15}$-producing *K. pneumoniae* K12-9 and the commensal *K. quasipneumoniae* MV91-24 isolates exhibited resistance to imipenem, thus indicating the wide dispersion of carbapenemases, either combined with ESBL or not, among different environments, a fact that has been described previously [42,43].

ESBL-producing *K. pneumoniae* can cause infection outbreaks in NICUs. In this study, some of the strains were isolated from blood cultures (*K. pneumoniae* K12-1 and K12-2), vascular catheters (*K. pneumoniae* K12-6), faeces (*K. michiganensis* K12-5 and K12-7 and *K. pneumoniae* K12-8, K12-9 and K12-10) or the environment (*K. variicola* K12-3 and *K. pneumoniae* K12-4) during the investigation of a neonatal-ICU outbreak. Most of them were MDR and ESBL-producing strains, despite the fact that they belonged to different *Klebsiella* species, thus suggesting the existence of a polyclonal outbreak in the NICU. The six *K. pneumoniae* isolates $bla_{CTX-M-15}$ producers, were grouped in three phylotypes (K12-1, K12-6 and K12-8; K12-4 and K12-9; K12-10), while the two MDR *K. michiganensis* isolates (K12-5 and K12-7) were not genetically related (Figure S1). Thus, although many outbreaks have been associated with the dissemination of a single clone, the polyclonal dissemination of different ESBL-producing *Klebsiella* strains can happen in the same unit at the same time [44]. Plasmids can play an essential role in the dissemination of antibiotic resistance among clinically relevant pathogens, as it has been described previously [44–46]. In this study, we have described that *Klebsiella* isolates possess a variable number (from 0 to 8) of large and small plasmids ranging from 1 to 600 kb in size which could reflects its ability to acquire and transfer genetic determinants, including virulence genes, pathogenicity islands and antimicrobial-resistance genes. The epidemiology of the NICU outbreak would require further investigation by using genomic approaches, as it was not the primary scope of this work.

The inverse correlation between antibiotic resistance and virulence has been previously proposed [47,48]. In this study, however, we did not find any correlation between antibiotic resistance and the carriage of virulence genes or the ability to produce biofilm or siderophores, despite a heterogeneity in the virulence factors being reported by other authors [37]. In the same manner, we did not observe strong correlations between the source of isolates (commensal, community acquired or NICU outbreak) and the presence of virulence traits. Similarly, little differences were found in the phenotypic and genomic characteristics of *Klebsiella* isolates recovered from healthy and sick infants [8].

None of the *Klebsiella* isolates harboured the *magA* and *rmpA* genes, which have been associated with the hypermucoviscosity phenotype in liver-invasive strains [26,27]. This was in agreement with the phenotypic assays performed in this work since none of the *Klebsiella* isolates studied showed a hypermucoviscous phenotype. In contrast, all members of the *K. pneumoniae* complex (with the exception of *K. pneumoniae* Ko9) presented the *fimH* gene encoding the type 1 fimbrial adhesion. Thus, 100% of commensal *K. pneumoniae* strains that were isolated from healthy subjects harboured the *fimH* gene, which is in contrast with the results of other authors, who found that *K. pneumoniae* strains isolated from the gut microbiota of healthy subjects were negative for that gene [10]. Other studies, however, have described a similar proportion of the *fimH* gene in *K. pneumoniae* isolates from community-acquired bacteraemia [27,37,49].

Within the *K. pneumoniae* complex, the *wabG* gene, encoding proteins involved in lipopolysaccharide synthesis [50] was detected in 38.2% of isolates and was more represented among commensal than among community-acquired isolates. Interestingly, the *wabG* gene was present in nearly all strains that had been isolated from faeces. The *uge* gene, encoding uridine diphosphate galacturonate 4-epimerase [51], was detected in 38.2% of isolates and was more abundant among the NICU outbreak isolates than among the community-acquired ones. In a recent study on *Klebsiella* spp. causing community-acquired infections, it has been described a positive rate of 28.2% and 61.5% for *wabG* and *uge* genes, respectively [37], while in other studies, the rates of positivity were close to 100% for both *uge* and *wabG* among virulent clones of *K. pneumoniae* [49,52]. Neither *wabG* nor *uge* were present in the isolates belonging to the *K. oxytoca* complex.

Iron is essential for the growth of most bacterial pathogens, so the ability to acquire iron is frequently associated with bacterial virulence. The *kfu* (iron-uptake system) gene has been associated with higher virulence in *K. pneumoniae* [26,53,54]. In our study, a low proportion of *K. pneumoniae* isolates carried the *kfu* gene, similarly as was recently described by other authors [10,37]. Interestingly, the two *K. variicola* strains (MV3-1 and K12-3) and *R. ornithinolytica* Ko10 presented the *kfu* gene. In addition, bacteria can obtain iron from the host by removing it via siderophore-mediated uptake systems. In our study, we designed a novel multiplex PCR to detect genes associated to biosynthesis or as receptors of the siderophores aerobactin (*iutA*, *iucB*), enterobactin (*fepA*, *fepC*) and yersibactin (*fyuA*, *ybtT*). Within the *K. pneumoniae* complex, the gene encoding enterobactin (*fepA*) was less abundant (64%) than the gene *fepC* encoding the receptor of enterobactin (79%). In addition, the enterobactin receptor gene (*fepC*) was more represented in commensal than in community-acquired isolates. In line with our results, recent studies have shown that enterobactin genes are present in a high proportion of the *K. pneumoniae* strains isolated from healthy and diseased preterm infants [8] and from community-acquired cases [37]. In relation to yersiniabactin, the synthesis (*fyuA*) and receptor (*ybtT*) genes were less represented than enterobactin-related genes, but all isolates harbouring the *fyuA* gene also presented the *ybtT* gene. In contrast, none of the isolates harboured the genes *iutA* and *iucB* encoding the synthesis and receptor genes of aerobactin. Those results agree with other studies were the yersiniabactin and aerobactin genes were less represented than those corresponding to enterobactin [10,37]. None of the *K. quasipneumoniae* isolates harboured any of the siderophores genes tested, while only one isolate of *K. variicola* harboured the gene encoding the enterobactin receptor.

Within the *K. oxytoca* complex, the *fepA* gene encoding enterobactin was not detected in any of the isolates, while the *fepC* gene encoding the enterobactin receptor was present in 55% of the isolates, all belonging to *K. michiganensis* strains. The gene encoding yersiniabactin (*fyuA*) was more represented in the *K. oxytoca* that in the *K. pneumoniae* complex and was only harboured by *K. michiganensis* and *K. grimontii*. However, all isolates harbouring the gene encoding yersiniabactin lacked the gene encoding its corresponding receptor (*ybtT*), which was only detected in *K. oxytoca* sensu stricto. Interestingly, the *fyuA* gene was less represented among community-acquired than among commensal isolates ($p < 0.05$). Aerobactin was not detected in any of the isolates of the *K. oxytoca* complex, while its receptor (*iucB*) was only detected in two *K. michiganensis* isolates. The genomic analysis of *K. michiganensis* and *K. grimontii* strains isolated from preterm infants has shown the presence of the enterobactin and yersiniabactin genes and the absence of the aerobactin gene in these species [8].

Our study has shown that most of *Klebsiella* isolates would be able to produce enterobactin, while a much smaller percentage would produce either aerobactin or yersiniabactin. Although these results agree with previous studies [1,8,10,37], our work revealed the high proportion of *Klebsiella* isolates that possess the gene encoding the receptor for enterobactin but not the gene for its biosynthesis. These isolates would be able to cheat the siderophore enterobactin produced by other bacteria, which could increase their competitiveness [55]. Finally, we did not find any correlation between the phenotypic production of siderophores and the presence of siderophore genes. This could be due to the presence of other iron-uptake systems different from that reported in this study, the lack of functionality of some of the genes studied by PCR or the existence of regulatory mechanisms, which would require further investigation.

The ability of the *Klebsiella* to produce antimicrobial compounds both in solid and liquid medium was also addressed in this work. Two isolates of *K. pneumoniae*, MV91-1 (commensal) and Kp5 (community-acquired), inhibited the growth of other *Klebsiella* strains when assayed on solid medium (Figure 4). The inhibitory activity of both strains was sensitive to proteinase K, thus indicating that they most likely produce bacteriocins, which are traditionally defined as antimicrobial compounds of proteinaceous nature with antimicrobial activity against related species [56]. The inhibitory spectrum of *K. pneumoniae* MV91-1 against the collection of *Klebsiella* isolates included in this work was extraordinarily wide, being active against *K. pneumoniae*, *K. quasipneumoniae* subsp. *similipneumoniae* and subsp. *quasipneumoniae*, *K. variicola*, *R. ornithinolytica*, *K. grimontii* and *K. michiganensis*. In contrast, the inhibitory spectrum of *K. pneumoniae* Kp5 was narrower, being active only against *K. pneumoniae*, *K. variicola* and *K. michiganensis*. Interestingly, both *K. pneumoniae* MV91-1 and Kp5 were active against all the MDR and ESBL-producing isolates from the NICU's outbreak. In addition, *K. pneumoniae* MV91-1 was active against the imipenem-resistant *K. pneumoniae* K12-9 and MV91-24 isolates. The characterization of these *K. pneumoniae* bacteriocins would open the door to the development of new antimicrobial strategies to combat *Klebsiella* strains, thus reducing the burden of antimicrobial resistance. In a recent study, it has been shown that bacteriocins from *Klebsiella* can be used for broad and efficient control of *Klebsiella* pathogens, in particular against MDR isolates [57].

The presence of different *Klebsiella* spp. in the milk of healthy women and in faeces of healthy breast-fed infants [15–17] suggest that these species are natural inhabitants of human microbiota, as has been described previously [8–13]. Attending to the virulence factors detected, the production of siderophores and biofilms and the plasmid content (small and large plasmids) observed, commensal strains were virtually indistinguishable from community-acquired and NICU outbreak isolates. Thus, these commensal isolates have all the potential to become pathogenic and cause infectious diseases, which is in line with the recent studies showing that many infections are self-acquired from the patient's own gastrointestinal microbiota [12,13]. The presence of virulence traits within each commensal strain could be determined by some of the conserved genes that form the core genome within each *Klebsiella* species, while other virulence and antibiotic resistance genes would be determined by a pool of accessory genes (accessory genome) that can be shared between different Klebsiella species and even between different genera [58]. Nowadays, it is becoming more evident that Klebsiella has the ability of exchanging and assembling a wide portfolio of genes that are involved in colonization, infection and antimicrobial resistance, which in the last instance would determine if a commensal strain remains asymptomatic or turns pathogenic [58]. Commensal Klebsiella isolates, which are well adapted to live and compete within the human microbiota, are prone to acquiring antibiotic resistant genes, by horizontal gene transfer, after the colonization with antibiotic-resistant Klebsiella strains acquired in hospital environments, such as an NICU, or from other host bacteria that have developed resistance after antibiotic treatments [59]. This combination (adaptation to the host and antibiotic resistance) could lead to the apparition of new MDR Klebsiella isolates that could be difficult to treat with current antibiotic-based strategies. This could be the case of the commensal isolate K. quapsineumoniae subsp. similipneumoniae MV91-42 (isolated from a healthy breast-fed infant) which is MDR, ESBL-producing and resistant to imipenem and that deserves further investigation.

Our results highlight the importance of studying Klebsiella spp. from the microbiota of healthy people, which could help to create surveillance programs aimed to know the prevalence of antibiotic resistance in the population. In this line, it has been proposed that the screening of the patient's gut microbiota after their admission to hospital could help to guide the application of the correct treatment [60]. Finally, we should increase our efforts in the development of novel alternatives or complementary strategies to antibiotics, which could help to reduce AMR in bacteria. These strategies could include the use of live biotherapeutic products, which has been demonstrated to be a real alternative to the use of antibiotics to combat infectious diseases [61] or the use of bacteriocins, such as plantaricin NC8 [62], as adjuvant in combination therapy to potentiate the effects of antibiotics and reduce their overall use [63]. The fact that the commensal isolate K. pneumoniae MV91-1 was able to inhibit the growth of the MDR, ESBL-producing, imipenem-resistant strains K12-9 and MV91-24, deserves to be further explored.

5. Conclusions

By sequencing a short region of the *rpoB* gene, we have determined that K. variicola and K. pseudoneumoniae isolates could be misidentified as K. pneumoniae by routine biochemical methods and that this biochemical misidentification is especially relevant within the K. oxytoca complex, where most isolates identified as K. oxytoca belong to K. michiganensis and, to a lesser extent, to K. grimontii and Raoultella species. Attending to the presence of virulence determinants, the production of siderophores or the ability to form biofilms, we were unable to distinguish between commensal Klebsiella strains isolated from healthy subjects and Klebsiella strains isolated from community-acquired infections or NICU nosocomial outbreaks. The only difference observed was the antibiotic susceptibility profiles since the strains isolated from the NICU's outbreak were ESBLs producers and harboured CTX-M-15 genes. Finally, while this study reveals that the human microbiota could constitute a reservoir of commensal Klebsiella isolates with the potential to become pathogenic, we have also demonstrated that it could be envisaged as a potential source of novel antimicrobials to combat the increasing threat of antibiotic resistance in Klebsiella spp.

Supplementary Materials: The following are available online at https://www.mdpi.com/article/10.3390/microorganisms9112344/s1, Figure S1: PFGE profiles of the isolates from the K. pneumoniae (A) and K. oxytoca complex (B), Figure S2: Plasmid profiles of isolates from K. pneumoniae (A) and K. oxytoca complex, Table S1: Oligonucleotides used in this study.

Author Contributions: Conceptualization, J.M.R. and A.M.-B.; methodology, M.G., A.V. and R.d.C.; software, R.d.C. and A.M.-B.; validation, M.G., A.V., J.M.R., R.d.C. and A.M.-B.; formal analysis, R.d.C., J.M.R. and A.M.-B.; investigation, M.G., A.V., R.d.C., J.M.R. and A.M.-B.; resources, R.d.C. and J.M.R.; data curation, A.M.-B.; writing—original draft preparation, A.M.-B.; writing—review and editing, M.G., A.V., R.d.C. and J.M.R.; supervision, J.M.R. and A.M.-B.; project administration,

J.M.R.; funding acquisition, J.M.R. All authors have read and agreed to the published version of the manuscript.

Funding: This research was funded by Ministerio de Ciencia e Innovación (Spain), grant numbers CSD2007-00063 (FUN-C-FOOD, Consolider-Ingenio 2010), AGL2010-15420 and PID2019-105606RB-I00.

Institutional Review Board Statement: The study was conducted according to the guidelines of the Declaration of Helsinki, and approved by the Ethical Committee of Clinical Research of the Hospital Clínico San Carlos (Madrid, Spain) (protocol code 10/017-E).

Informed Consent Statement: Informed consent was obtained from all subjects involved in the study.

Data Availability Statement: The *rpoB* gene sequences obtained in this study were deposited in the GenBank database, under the accession numbers KJ499842 to KJ499903.

Acknowledgments: We would like to express our gratitude to Fernando Cháves, the research group UCM 920080 and the departments of Microbiology of the hospitals Doce de Octubre and Ramón y Cajal (Madrid, Spain) for providing us with the *Klebsiella* isolates used in this work.

Conflicts of Interest: The authors declare no conflict of interest. The funders had no role in the design of the study; in the collection, analyses, or interpretation of data; in the writing of the manuscript, or in the decision to publish the results.

References

1. Podschun, R.; Ullmann, U. *Klebsiella* spp. as nosocomial pathogens: Epidemiology, taxonomy, typing methods, and pathogenicity factors. *Clin. Microbiol. Rev.* **1998**, *11*, 589–603. [CrossRef] [PubMed]
2. Bengoechea, J.A.; Sa Pessoa, J. *Klebsiella pneumoniae* infection biology: Living to counteract host defences. *FEMS Microbiol. Rev.* **2019**, *43*, 123–144. [CrossRef]
3. Blin, C.; Passet, V.; Touchon, M.; Rocha, E.P.C.; Brisse, S. Metabolic diversity of the emerging pathogenic lineages of *Klebsiella pneumoniae*. *Environ. Microbiol.* **2017**, *19*, 1881–1898. [CrossRef]
4. Brisse, S.; Verhoef, J. Phylogenetic diversity of *Klebsiella pneumoniae* and *Klebsiella oxytoca* clinical isolates revealed by randomly amplified polymorphic DNA, *gyr*A and *par*C genes sequencing and automated ribotyping. *Int. J. Syst. Evol. Microbiol.* **2001**, *51*, 915–924. [CrossRef]
5. Rodrigues, C.; Passet, V.; Rakotondrasoa, A.; Diallo, T.A.; Criscuolo, A.; Brisse, S. Description of *Klebsiella africanensis* sp. nov., *Klebsiella variicola* subsp. *tropicalensis* subsp. nov. and *Klebsiella variicola* subsp. *variicola* subsp. nov. *Res. Microbiol.* **2019**, *170*, 165–170. [CrossRef]
6. Merla, C.; Rodrigues, C.; Passet, V.; Corbella, M.; Thorpe, H.A.; Kallonen, T.V.S.; Zong, Z.; Marone, P.; Bandi, C.; Sassera, D.; et al. Description of *Klebsiella spallanzanii* sp. nov. and of *Klebsiella pasteurii* sp. nov. *Front. Microbiol.* **2019**, *10*, 2360. [CrossRef]
7. Long, S.W.; Linson, S.E.; Ojeda Saavedra, M.; Cantu, C.; Davis, J.J.; Brettin, T.; Olsen, R.J. Whole-genome sequencing of human clinical *Klebsiella pneumoniae* isolates reveals misidentification and misunderstandings of *Klebsiella pneumoniae, Klebsiella variicola*, and *Klebsiella quasipneumoniae*. *mSphere* **2017**, *2*, e00290-17. [CrossRef]
8. Chen, Y.; Brook, T.C.; Soe, C.Z.; O'Neill, I.; Alcon-Giner, C.; Leelastwattanagul, O.; Phillips, S.; Caim, S.; Clarke, P.; Hall, L.J.; et al. Preterm infants harbour diverse *Klebsiella* populations, including atypical species that encode and produce an array of antimicrobial resistance- and virulence-associated factors. *Microb. Genom.* **2020**, *6*, e000377. [CrossRef] [PubMed]
9. Conlan, S.; Kong, H.H.; Segre, J.A. Species-level analysis of DNA sequence data from the NIH Human Microbiome Project. *PLoS ONE* **2012**, *7*, e47075. [CrossRef] [PubMed]
10. Amaretti, A.; Righini, L.; Candeliere, F.; Musmeci, E.; Bonvicini, F.; Gentilomi, G.A.; Rossi, M.; Raimondi, S. Antibiotic resistance, virulence factors, phenotyping, and genotyping of non-*Escherichia coli* Enterobacterales from the gut microbiota of healthy subjects. *Int. J. Mol. Sci.* **2020**, *21*, 1847. [CrossRef]
11. Chung, D.R.; Lee, H.; Park, M.H.; Jung, S.I.; Chang, H.H.; Kim, Y.S.; Son, J.S.; Moon, C.; Kwon, K.T.; Ryu, S.Y.; et al. Fecal carriage of serotype K1 *Klebsiella pneumoniae* ST23 strains closely related to liver abscess isolates in Koreans living in Korea. *Eur. J. Clin. Microbiol. Infect. Dis.* **2012**, *31*, 481–486. [CrossRef] [PubMed]
12. Gorrie, C.L.; Mirceta, M.; Wick, R.R.; Edwards, D.J.; Thomson, N.R.; Strugnell, R.A.; Pratt, N.F.; Garlick, J.S.; Watson, K.M.; Pilcher, D.V.; et al. Gastrointestinal carriage is a major reservoir of *Klebsiella pneumoniae* infection in intensive care patients. *Clin. Infect. Dis.* **2017**, *65*, 208–215. [CrossRef] [PubMed]
13. Martin, R.M.; Cao, J.; Brisse, S.; Passet, V.; Wu, W.; Zhao, L.; Malani, P.N.; Rao, K.; Bachman, M.A. Molecular epidemiology of colonizing and infecting isolates of *Klebsiella pneumoniae*. *mSphere* **2016**, *1*, e00261-16. [CrossRef]
14. Clark, R.; Powers, R.; White, R.; Bloom, B.; Sanchez, P.; Benjamin, D.K., Jr. Nosocomial infection in the NICU: A medical complication or unavoidable problem? *J. Perinatol.* **2004**, *24*, 382–388. [CrossRef] [PubMed]
15. Fernández, L.; Langa, S.; Martín, V.; Maldonado, A.; Jiménez, E.; Martín, R.; Rodríguez, J.M. The human milk microbiota: Origin and potential roles in health and disease. *Pharmacol. Res.* **2013**, *69*, 1–10. [CrossRef] [PubMed]

16. Rodríguez-Cruz, M.; Alba, C.; Aparicio, M.; Checa, M.Á.; Fernández, L.; Rodríguez, J.M. Effect of sample collection (manual expression vs. pumping) and skimming on the microbial profile of human milk using culture techniques and metataxonomic analysis. *Microorganisms* **2020**, *8*, 1278. [CrossRef]
17. Martín, V.; Maldonado, A.; Rodríguez-Baños, M.; del Campo, R.; Rodríguez, J.M.; Jiménez, E. Sharing of bacterial strains between breast milk and infant faeces. *J. Hum. Lact.* **2012**, *28*, 36–44. [CrossRef] [PubMed]
18. Thompson, J.D.; Higgins, D.G.; Gibson, T.J. CLUSTAL W: Improving the sensitivity of progressive multiple sequence alignment through sequence weighting, position-specific gap penalties and weight matrix choice. *Nucleic Acids Res.* **1994**, *22*, 4673. [CrossRef]
19. Tamura, K.; Stecher, G.; Peterson, D.; Filipski, A.; Kumar, S. MEGA6: Molecular Evolutionary Genetics Analysis version 6.0. *Mol. Biol. Evol.* **2013**, *30*, 2725–2729. [CrossRef]
20. Saitou, N.; Nei, M. The neighbor-joining method: A new method for reconstructing phylogenetic trees. *Mol. Biol. Evol.* **1987**, *4*, 406–425.
21. Kaufmann, M.E. Pulsed-field gel electrophoresis. In *Molecular Bacteriology: Protocols and Clinical Applications*; Woodford, N., Johnson, A.P., Eds.; Humana Press: Totowa, NJ, USA, 1998; pp. 33–50.
22. Jarlier, V.; Nicolas, M.-H.; Fournier, G.; Philippon, A. Extended broad-spectrum β-lactamases conferring transferable resistance to newer β-lactam agents in Enterobacteriaceae: Hospital prevalence and susceptibility pattern. *Rev. Infect. Dis.* **1988**, *10*, 867–878. [CrossRef]
23. Woodford, N.; Fagan, E.J.; Ellington, M.J. Multiplex PCR for rapid detection of genes encoding CTX-M extended-spectrum (beta)-lactamases. *J. Antimicrob. Chemother.* **2006**, *57*, 154–155. [CrossRef] [PubMed]
24. Wang, H.; Kelkar, S.; Wu, W.; Chen, M.; Quinn, J.I. Clinical isolates of Enterobacteriaceae producing extended-spectrum beta-lactamases: Prevalence of CTX-M-3 at a hospital in China. *Antimicrob. Agents Chemother.* **2003**, *47*, 790–793. [CrossRef] [PubMed]
25. Magiorakos, A.P.; Srinivasan, A.; Carey, R.B.; Carmeli, Y.; Falagas, M.E.; Giske, C.G.; Harbarth, S.; Hindler, J.F.; Kahlmeter, G.; Olsson-Liljequist, B.; et al. Multidrug-resistant, extensively drug-resistant and pandrug-resistant bacteria: An international expert proposal for interim standard definitions for acquired resistance. *Clin. Microbiol. Infect.* **2012**, *18*, 268–281. [CrossRef]
26. Fang, C.T.; Chuang, Y.P.; Shun, C.T.; Chang, S.C.; Wang, J.T. A novel virulence gene in *Klebsiella pneumoniae* strains causing primary liver abscess and septic metastatic complications. *J. Exp. Med.* **2004**, *199*, 697–705. [CrossRef]
27. Yu, W.L.; Ko, W.C.; Cheng, K.C.; Lee, H.C.; Ke, D.S.; Lee, C.C.; Fung, C.P.; Chuang, Y.C. Association between *rmp*A and *mag*A genes and clinical syndromes caused by *Klebsiella pneumoniae* in Taiwan. *Clin. Infect. Dis.* **2006**, *42*, 1351–1358. [CrossRef] [PubMed]
28. Shon, A.S.; Bajwa, R.P.; Russo, T.A. Hypervirulent (hypermucoviscous) *Klebsiella pneumoniae*: A new and dangerous breed. *Virulence* **2013**, *4*, 107–118. [CrossRef] [PubMed]
29. Fletcher, M. Adhesion and biofilm development of acetate-, propionate-, and butyrate-degrading microorganisms on glass surfaces. *Can. J. Microbiol.* **1977**, *23*, 1–6. [CrossRef]
30. O'Toole, G.A.; Kolter, R. Initiation of biofilm formation in *Pseudomonas fluorescens* WCS365 proceeds via multiple, convergent signalling pathways: A genetic analysis. *Mol. Microbiol.* **1998**, *28*, 449–461. [CrossRef] [PubMed]
31. Schwyn, B.; Neilands, J.B. Universal chemical assay for the detection and determination of siderophores. *Anal. Biochem.* **1987**, *160*, 47–56. [CrossRef]
32. Tagg, J.R.; Dajani, A.S.; Wannamaker, L.W. Bacteriocins of Gram-positive bacteria. *Bacteriol. Rev.* **1976**, *40*, 722–756. [CrossRef]
33. Harris, L.J.; Daescheyl, M.A.; Stiles, M.E.; Klaenhammer, T.R. Antimicrobial activity of lactic acid bacteria against *Listeria monocytogenes*. *J. Food Prot.* **1999**, *52*, 384–887. [CrossRef]
34. European Centre for Disease Prevention and Control. *Antimicrobial Resistance in the EU/EEA (EARS-Net)—Annual Epidemiological Report 2019*; ECDC: Stockholm, Sweden, 2020.
35. Boye, K.; Hansen, D.S. Sequencing of 16S rDNA of *Klebsiella*: Taxonomic relations within the genus and to other Enterobacteriaceae. *Int. J. Med. Microbiol.* **2003**, *292*, 495–503. [CrossRef] [PubMed]
36. Drancourt, M.; Bollet, C.; Carta, A.; Rousselier, P. Phylogenetic analyses of *Klebsiella* species delineate *Klebsiella* and *Raoultella* gen. nov., with description of *Raoultella ornithinolytica* comb. nov., *Raoultella terrigena* comb. nov. and *Raoultella planticola* comb. nov. *Int. J. Syst. Evol. Microbiol.* **2001**, *51*, 925–932. [CrossRef] [PubMed]
37. Garza-Ramos, U.; Barrios-Camacho, H.; Moreno-Domínguez, S.; Toribio-Jiménez, J.; Jardón-Pineda, D.; Cuevas-Peña, J.; Sánchez-Pérez, A.; Duran-Bedolla, J.; Olguín-Rodriguez, J.; Román-Román, A. Phenotypic and molecular characterization of *Klebsiella* spp. isolates causing community-acquired infections. *New Microbes New Infect.* **2018**, *23*, 17–27. [CrossRef]
38. Hajjar, R.; Ambaraghassi, G.; Sebajang, H.; Schwenter, F.; Su, S.H. *Raoultella ornithinolytica*: Emergence and resistance. *Infect. Drug Resist.* **2020**, *13*, 1091–1104. [CrossRef] [PubMed]
39. Mehmood, H.; Pervin, N.; Israr Ul Haq, M.; Kamal, K.R.; Marwat, A.; Khan, M. A rare case of *Raoultella planticola* urinary tract infection in a patient with immunoglobulin a nephropathy. *J. Investig. Med. High Impact Case Rep.* **2018**, *6*, 2324709618780422.
40. Chapman, P.; Forde, B.M.; Roberts, L.W.; Bergh, H.; Vesey, D.; Jennison, A.V.; Moss, S.; Paterson, D.L.; Beatson, S.A.; Harris, P.N.A. Genomic Investigation reveals contaminated detergent as the source of an extended-spectrum-β-lactamase-producing *Klebsiella michiganensis* outbreak in a neonatal unit. *J. Clin. Microbiol.* **2020**, *58*, e01980-19. [CrossRef]
41. Rodríguez-Medina, N.; Barrios-Camacho, H.; Duran-Bedolla, J.; Garza-Ramos, U. *Klebsiella variicola*: An emerging pathogen in humans. *Emerg. Microbes Infect.* **2019**, *8*, 973–988. [CrossRef]

42. Perdigão, J.; Caneiras, C.; Elias, R.; Modesto, A.; Spadar, A.; Phelan, J.; Campino, S.; Clark, T.G.; Costa, E.; Saavedra, M.J.; et al. Genomic epidemiology of carbapenemase producing *Klebsiella pneumoniae* strains at a northern Portuguese hospital enables the detection of a misidentified *Klebsiella variicola* KPC-3 producing strain. *Microorganisms* **2020**, *8*, 1986. [CrossRef]
43. Nordmann, P.; Cuzon, G.; Naas, T. The real threat of *Klebsiella pneumoniae* carbapenemase-producing bacteria. *Lancet Infect. Dis.* **2009**, *9*, 228–236. [CrossRef]
44. Fiett, J.; Palucha, A.; Miaczynska, B.; Stankiewicz, M.; Przondo-Mordarska, H.; Hryniewicz, W.; Gniadkowski, M. A novel complex mutant beta-lactamase, TEM-68, identified in a *Klebsiella pneumoniae* isolate from an outbreak of extended-spectrum beta-lactamase-producing *Klebsiellae*. *Antimicrob. Agents Chemother.* **2000**, *44*, 1499–1505. [CrossRef]
45. Bingen, E.H.; Desjardins, P.; Arlet, G.; Bourgeois, F.; Mariani-Kurkdjian, P.; Lambert-Zechovsky, N.Y.; Denamur, E.; Philippon, A.; Elion, J. Molecular epidemiology of plasmid spread among extended broad-spectrum beta-lactamase-producing *Klebsiella pneumoniae* isolates in a pediatric hospital. *J. Clin. Microbiol.* **1993**, *31*, 179–184. [CrossRef] [PubMed]
46. San Millan, A. Evolution of plasmid-mediated antibiotic resistance in the clinical context. *Trends Microbiol.* **2018**, *26*, 978–985. [CrossRef] [PubMed]
47. Hennequin, C.; Robin, F. Correlation between antimicrobial resistance and virulence in *Klebsiella pneumoniae*. *Eur. J. Clin. Microbiol. Infect. Dis.* **2016**, *35*, 333–341. [CrossRef]
48. Beceiro, A.; Tomás, M.; Bou, G. Antimicrobial resistance and virulence: A successful or deleterious association in the bacterial world? *Clin. Microbiol. Rev.* **2013**, *26*, 185–230. [CrossRef] [PubMed]
49. Brisse, S.; Fevre, C.; Passet, V.; Issenhuth-Jeanjean, S.; Tournebize, R.; Diancourt, L.; Grimont, P. Virulent clones of *Klebsiella pneumoniae*: Identification and evolutionary scenario based on genomic and phenotypic characterization. *PLoS ONE* **2009**, *4*, e4982. [CrossRef]
50. Izquierdo, L.; Coderch, N.; Piqué, N.; Bedini, E.; Corsaro, M.M.; Merino, S.; Fresno, S.; Tomas, J.M.; Regué, M. The *Klebsiella pneumoniae* wabG gene: Role in biosynthesis of the core lipopolysaccharide and virulence. *J. Bacteriol.* **2003**, *185*, 7213–7221. [CrossRef]
51. Regué, M.; Hita, B.; Piqué, N.; Izquierdo, L.; Merino, S.; Fresno, S.; Benedí, V.J.; Tomás, J.M. A gene, *uge*, is essential for *Klebsiella pneumoniae* virulence. *Infect. Immun.* **2004**, *72*, 54–61. [CrossRef]
52. Fursova, N.K.; Astashkin, E.I.; Ershova, O.N.; Aleksandrova, I.A.; Savin, I.A.; Novikova, T.S.; Fedyukina, G.N.; Kislichkina, A.A.; Fursov, M.V.; Kuzina, E.S.; et al. Multidrug-resistant *Klebsiella pneumoniae* causing severe infections in the neuro-ICU. *Antibiotics* **2021**, *10*, 979. [CrossRef]
53. Ma, L.C.; Fang, C.T.; Lee, C.Z.; Shun, C.T.; Wang, J.T. Genomic heterogeneity in *Klebsiella pneumoniae* strains is associated with primary pyogenic liver abscess and metastatic infection. *J. Infect. Dis.* **2005**, *192*, 117–128. [CrossRef] [PubMed]
54. Dogan, O.; Vatansever, C.; Atac, N.; Albayrak, O.; Karahuseyinoglu, S.; Sahin, O.E.; Kilicoglu, B.K.; Demiray, A.; Ergonul, O.; Gönen, M.; et al. Virulence determinants of colistin-resistant *K. pneumoniae* high-risk clones. *Biology (Basel)* **2021**, *10*, 436. [CrossRef] [PubMed]
55. Kramer, J.; Özkaya, Ö.; Kümmerli, R. Bacterial siderophores in community and host interactions. *Nat. Rev. Microbiol.* **2020**, *18*, 152–163. [CrossRef] [PubMed]
56. Cotter, P.D.; Hill, C.; Ross, R.P. Bacteriocins: Developing innate immunity for food. *Nat. Rev. Microbiol.* **2005**, *3*, 777–788. [CrossRef] [PubMed]
57. Denkovskienė, E.; Paškevičius, Š.; Misiūnas, A.; Stočkūnaitė, B.; Starkevič, U.; Vitkauskienė, A.; Hahn-Löbmann, S.; Schulz, S.; Giritch, A.; Gleba, Y.; et al. Broad and efficient control of *Klebsiella* pathogens by peptidoglycan-degrading and pore-forming bacteriocins klebicins. *Sci. Rep.* **2019**, *9*, 15422. [CrossRef]
58. Martin, R.M.; Bachman, M.A. Colonization, Infection, and the Accessory Genome of Klebsiella pneumoniae. *Front. Cell. Infect. Microbiol.* **2018**, *8*, 4. [CrossRef]
59. Ghenea, A.E.; Cioboată, R.; Drocaş, A.I.; Ţieranu, E.N.; Vasile, C.M.; Moroşanu, A.; Ţieranu, C.G.; Salan, A.-I.; Popescu, M.; Turculeanu, A.; et al. Prevalence and Antimicrobial Resistance of Klebsiella Strains Isolated from a County Hospital in Romania. *Antibiotics* **2021**, *10*, 868. [CrossRef]
60. Dorman, M.J.; Short, F.L. Genome watch: *Klebsiella pneumoniae*: When a colonizer turns bad. *Nat. Rev. Microbiol.* **2017**, *15*, 384. [CrossRef]
61. Arroyo, R.; Martín, V.; Maldonado, A.; Jiménez, E.; Fernández, L.; Rodríguez, J.M. Treatment of infectious mastitis during lactation: Antibiotics versus oral administration of Lactobacilli isolated from breast milk. *Clin. Infect. Dis.* **2010**, *50*, 1551–1558. [CrossRef]
62. Maldonado, A.; Ruiz-Barba, J.L.; Jiménez-Díaz, R. Purification and genetic characterization of plantaricin NC8, a novel coculture-inducible two-peptide bacteriocin from *Lactobacillus plantarum* NC8. *Appl. Environ. Microbiol.* **2003**, *69*, 383–389. [CrossRef]
63. Bengtsson, T.; Selegård, R.; Musa, A.; Hultenby, K.; Utterström, J.; Sivlér, P.; Skog, M.; Nayeri, F.; Hellmark, B.; Söderquist, B.; et al. Plantaricin NC8 $\alpha\beta$ exerts potent antimicrobial activity against *Staphylococcus* spp. and enhances the effects of antibiotics. *Sci. Rep.* **2020**, *10*, 3580. [CrossRef] [PubMed]

Outer Membrane Protein F Is Involved in Biofilm Formation, Virulence and Antibiotic Resistance in *Cronobacter sakazakii*

Jianxin Gao [1], Zhonghui Han [2], Ping Li [3], Hongyan Zhang [1], Xinjun Du [3,*] and Shuo Wang [4,*]

1. Key Laboratory of Animal Resistance Biology of Shandong Province, Key Laboratory of Food Nutrition and Safety, School of Life Science, Shandong Normal University, Jinan 250014, China; jxgao@sdnu.edu.cn (J.G.); zhanghongyan@sdnu.edu.cn (H.Z.)
2. School of Food Science and Engineering, Qilu University of Technology, Shandong Academy of Sciences, Jinan 250353, China; zhhan@qlu.edu.cn
3. School of Food Science and Engineering, Tianjin University of Science and Technology, Tianjin 300457, China; zoelxx@tust.edu.cn
4. Tianjin Key Laboratory of Food Science and Health, School of Medicine, Nankai University, Tianjin 300071, China
* Correspondence: xjdu@tust.edu.cn (X.D.); wangshuo@nankai.edu.cn (S.W.)

Abstract: In some Gram-negative bacteria, *ompF* encodes outer membrane protein F (OmpF), which is a cation-selective porin and is responsible for the passive transport of small molecules across the outer membrane. However, there are few reports about the functions of this gene in *Cronobacter sakazakii*. To investigate the role of *ompF* in detail, an *ompF* disruption strain (Δ*ompF*) and a complementation strain (cp*ompF*) were successfully obtained. We find that OmpF can affect the ability of biofilm formation in *C. sakazakii*. In addition, the variations in biofilm composition of *C. sakazakii* were examined using Raman spectroscopy analyses caused by knocking out *ompF*, and the result indicated that the levels of certain biofilm components, including lipopolysaccharide (LPS), were significantly decreased in the mutant (Δ*ompF*). Then, SDS-PAGE was used to further analyze the LPS content, and the result showed that the LPS levels were significantly reduced in the absence of *ompF*. Therefore, we conclude that OmpF affects biofilm formation in *C. sakazakii* by reducing the amount of LPS. Furthermore, the Δ*ompF* mutant showed decreased (2.7-fold) adhesion to and invasion of HCT-8 cells. In an antibiotic susceptibility analysis, the Δ*ompF* mutant showed significantly smaller inhibition zones than the WT, indicating that OmpF had a positive effect on the influx of antibiotics into the cells. In summary, *ompF* plays a positive regulatory role in the biofilm formation and adhesion/invasion, which is achieved by regulating the amount of LPS, but is a negative regulator of antibiotic resistance in *C. sakazakii*.

Keywords: *ompF*; *Cronobacter sakazakii*; LPS; biofilm formation; adhesion/invasion

1. Introduction

Cronobacter sakazakii is an opportunistic food-borne pathogen that is associated with outbreaks of life-threatening bacteremia, meningitis and necrotizing enterocolitis (NEC) in neonates and infants, with case fatality rates reported to be as high as 40–80% and survivors frequently left with severe neurological and developmental disorders [1,2]. In addition, while not only causing newborn disease, *C. sakazaki* also infects adults. *C. sakazakii* CC4 and *C. sakazakii* ST12 have been recognized as specific pathovars associated with particular neonatal and adult infections [3,4]. In addition, *C. sakazakii* also has a wide range of habitats, and it has been found in powdered milk substitutes, meters and even in domestic kitchen sponges [5–7].

C. sakazakii strains have the capacity to invade and translocate through the Caco-2 and human brain microvascular endothelial cell lines [8]. These organisms can form biofilms, which can adhere to substrate surfaces, survive in the presence of antibiotics and disinfectants and enhance the resistance of cells to environmental stress [9]. In addition, Lehner and Kim reported that *Cronobacter* spp. have the ability to form biofilms to enhance adherence and improve pathogenesis [10,11]. Hartmann et al. suggested that the hypothetical proteins ESA_00281 and ESA_00282 have a strong impact on biofilm formation and contribute to the adhesion of *C. sakazakii* to Caco-2 intestinal epithelial cells [12]. In our previous work, using a random transposon insertion mutant library, we showed that the interactions of the *ompF* gene was mostly associated with biofilm formation in *C. sakazakii*. Therefore, it is reasonable to speculate that the *ompF* gene plays a vital role in the pathogenesis of *C. sakazakii*. However, there is very little information about how this gene works exactly on the biofilm-related pathogenesis of *C. sakazakii*.

Several outer membrane porin proteins (OMPs) have been discovered in Gram-negative bacteria; these proteins are β-barrel integral membrane proteins that form non-specific water-filled channels, allowing the passive diffusion of ions and molecules with molecular masses up to 600 Da [13,14]. OmpF is one of the most abundant proteins found in the outer membranes (OMs) of Gram-negative bacteria [15,16]. Prehna et al. demonstrated that OmpF and outer membrane protein C (OmpC) not only function to import ions and protein toxins but also contribute to the export of YebF, a 10.8 kDa soluble endogenous protein, in *E. coli* [17]. In addition, Nicholas et al. reported that an intrinsically disordered protein could tunnel through OmpF to deliver an epitope signal to the cell and initiate cell death. Additionally, OmpF can also serve as an entryway into cells for many antibiotics [18,19]. However, the function of *ompF* in *C. sakazakii* is still unclear. In this study, we generated an *ompF* deletion mutant (Δ*ompF*) and complementation controls in *C. sakazakii* ATCC BAA-894 to investigate the function of this gene. The biofilm formation ability was estimated, and the differences in the biochemical components of the biofilms of the different *C. sakazakii* ATCC BAA-894 strains were analyzed. Meanwhile, the ability of the *C. sakazakii* strains to invade or adhere to HCT-8 cells was investigated by an invasion/adhesion assay. In addition, we studied the difference in cell permeability and antibiotic resistance between the *C. sakazakii* ATCC BAA-894 wild_type and mutant strains. The research aim was to demonstrate the role of the *ompF* homolog of *C. sakazakii* ATCC BAA-894 in virulence and permeability.

2. Materials and Methods

2.1. Bacterial Strains, Plasmids and Culture Conditions

All the bacterial strains and plasmids used in this study are listed in Table S1. *Cronobacter sakazakii* and *Escherichia coli* were incubated on Luria–Bertani (LB; Difco, MD, USA) at 37 °C with constant shaking at 200 rpm. When needed, kanamycin, chloramphenicol or ampicillin was used at final concentrations of 100 µg/mL, 10 µg/mL and 100 µg/mL, respectively.

2.2. Construction of ompF Deletion Mutant

We constructed an *ompF* mutant using the Lambda-Red recombination system according to procedures reported by Kim et al. [20]. Briefly, using pET-26b plasmid as a template and KF/KR as primers, the kanamycin resistance cassette was amplified by PCR. Then, after digesting with *Bam*HI and *Sal*I, the PCR product was cloned into the pMD18-T vector to generate pMDK. The upstream and downstream flanking regions of the *ompF* gene were amplified with the two primer pairs 413UF/413UR and 413DF/413DR using the genomic DNA of *C. sakazakii* ATCC BAA-894 as template; the whole-genome sequence was obtained from GenBank. Then, the upstream DNA fragment of *ompF* was digested with *Kpn*I and *Bam*HI and inserted into the corresponding sites of pMDK to yield pMDKU. Then, both the downstream DNA fragment of *ompF* and the pMDKU plasmid were digested with *Sal*I and *Hind*III and then ligated by T4 DNA ligase to generate the plasmid pMDKUD, which was then transformed into *E. coli* DH5α. The *ompF*-upstream-kana-*ompF*-downstream product double digested with restriction endonucleases was transformed via electroporation into *C. sakazakii* ATCC BAA-894 (the wild_type, WT) harboring the pKD46 plasmid. Kanamycin-resistant transformants were selected to further verify successful mutation (Δ*ompF*). The sequences of all primers used are listed in Table S2.

2.3. Complementation Study

The complement plasmid pACYC184-*ompF*, which contains the *ompF* gene sequence and the native promoter, was constructed. The *ompF* sequence was amplified from wild_type *C. sakazakii* ATCC BAA-894 genomic DNA using the primer pair *ompF*-pACYC-F/*ompF*-pACYC-R (restriction enzyme sites *Bam*HI and *Sal*I were introduced into the primers). The PCR product was digested with the restriction endonucleases *Bam*HI and *Sal*I and cloned into the pACYC184 plasmid. Subsequently, the recombinant plasmid (pACYC184-ompF) was transferred into the Δ*ompF* mutant to generate the *ompF* complementation strain (cp*ompF*) [21]. Nucleotide sequencing was performed to confirm that the *ompF* coding region was in the pACYC184-*ompF*.

2.4. Growth Curves

The growth curve was interpreted by measuring the concentration of bacteria at different times by an ultraviolet spectrophotometer. The *C. sakazakii* strains ATCC BAA-894, Δ*ompF* and cp*ompF* inocula were cultured at 37 °C overnight without shaking in LB solid medium, and then subcultured in 50 mL of LB liquid medium at a ratio of 1:100. The cultures were incubated at 37 °C for 14 h with shaking at 200 rpm. The optical density at a wavelength of 600 nm (OD_{600}) was measured every hour. Samples with excessive concentrations ($OD_{600} > 0.8$) were diluted before measurement and the final OD_{600} value was calculated by multiplying the dilution factor by the OD_{600} value of the diluted bacterial solution.

2.5. Morphological Differences

Scanning electron microscopy (SEM, Hitachi, Japan) was employed to observe the morphological differences among WT, Δ*ompF* and cp*ompF* strains. All the strains were collected by centrifugation in the logarithmic phase of growth. Following washing with phosphate-buffered saline (0.1 mmol/L) 2 times, the strains of BAA-894 (wild type), mutant and complementation were fixed with glutaraldehyde (2.5%, wt/vol) at 4 °C for 24 h, respectively. Then, the cells were rinsed with distilled water 3 times and fixed with osmium tetroxide (1%) for 1 h, which was followed by dehydration for 10 min with a series of alcohol (25–100%). The bacteria were further freeze-dried under vacuum for 4 h. Finally, SEM was used to examine the dehydrated bacterial powder using an accelerating voltage of 5 kV.

2.6. Analysis of Biofilm Formation Ability

The ability of biofilm formation was performed with cultures grown in 96-well polystyrene plates using crystal violet staining according to the method developed by Hu Lan with some modifications [22]. The *C. sakazakii* strains were inoculated overnight on LB at 37 °C with shaking (200 rpm). Then, the strains were transferred into 7 mL fresh medium (1:100 dilution) and grown until the cells reached the logarithmic period. Two hundred-microliter aliquots were added in triplicate into 96-well plates, and the plates were incubated at 37 °C for 48 h without shaking. The plates were gently rinsed 3 times with sterile PBS, and the adherent bacterial cells were fixed with 200 µL of 99% methanol for 15 min. Then, the plates were air-dried and stained with 200 µL of 0.1% crystal violet (CV) for 30 min at room temperature. After rinsing 3 times with distilled water, the CV bound to the biofilm was released with 200 µL of 95% ethanol for 20 min. The absorbance was determined at 570 nm by a Sunrise Basic microplate reader (Tecan, Austria). The biofilm assay was performed in three separate experiments for each strain.

2.7. Determination of Biofilm Biochemical Components

Biofilm biochemical components in *Cronobacter sakazakii* were determined by Raman spectroscopy analyses and the same methods as in our previous work [23].

2.8. Analysis of C. sakazakii LPS by SDS-Polyacrylamide Gel Electrophoresis (SDS-PAGE)

To investigate the function of *ompF* in *C. sakazakii* ATCC BAA-894 (WT), Δ*ompF* and cp*ompF* strains, the LPS was extracted from strains WT, Δ*ompF* and cp*ompF*, using the modified hot phenol–water method reported by Hong et al. [24]. Briefly, WT, Δ*ompF* and cp*ompF* strains were cultured overnight on LB medium at 37 °C and subcultured as a 1% overnight culture in 100 mL of LB medium. After the strain was cultured to 10^8 CFU/mL, 100 mL of each cell suspension was added to an equal volume of 45% phenol solution for 5 min, and then an equal volume of 95% phenol solution was added with vigorous stirring for 20–30 min at 68 °C. When the solution cooled to about 10 °C, it was centrifuged at $5000 \times g$ for 45 min at 10 °C. The LPS was fractionated in the upper aqueous phase, and residual phenol was removed by dialyzing against water to obtain crude LPS. The LPS was further extracted with DNase I, RNaseA and proteinase K to eliminate contaminants. The purified LPS was finally precipitated with acetone. The LPS samples were subjected by SDS-polyacrylamide gel electrophoresis (SDS-PAGE) using a 5% (wt/vol) stacking gel and a 15% (wt/vol) resolving gel, which was followed by silver staining [25]. The images were visualized and photographed with a Molecular Imager Gel Doc^{TM} XR$^+$ (Bio-Rad Laboratories, Inc., Hercules, CA, USA).

2.9. Adhesion/Invasion Assay

An invasion assay on the *C. sakazakii* strain was conducted following a modified method of Rogers et al. to determine the adhesion/invasion of the bacteria [26]. HCT-8 cells (ATCC CCL-244, Manassas, Virginia) were cultured in RPMI 1640 (Invitrogen, Carlsbad, CA, USA) containing 10% (vol/vol) fetal bovine serum (FBS, Invitrogen, Waltham, MA, USA) at 37 °C and 5% CO_2. *C. sakazakii* strains were grown overnight at 37 °C in aerobic conditions, and then overnight cultures of *C. sakazakii* were transferred into fresh LB medium. The *C. sakazakii* cells were harvested by centrifugation (at $3000 \times g$ for 5 min at 4 °C) and then washed twice and resuspended with RPMI 1640. For the invasion assays, the *C. sakazakii* cells in RPMI 1640 were added onto washed HCT-8 cells that were >90% confluent (approximately 1×10^8 CFU/well) in 6-well tissue culture plates, giving a multiplicity of infection (MOI) of 100. After incubating for 3 h in the presence of 5% CO_2, the tissue culture plates were gently washed 3 times with PBS to remove nonattached bacteria. One milliliter of 0.1% Triton X-100 was added to each well to lyse the cells for 10 min. Finally, dilutions were plated onto plate count agar (PCA) to enumerate the CFU. All experiments shown were performed at least 3 times with a minimum of duplicate wells in each experiment.

2.10. Cell Permeability Assay

The *C. sakazakii* ATCC BAA-894 (wild type), Δ*ompF* and cp*ompF* strains in the log phase of growth were centrifuged at $3000 \times g$ for 10 min and incubated for 3 h in PBS containing 100 μg/mL arginine or lysine. The strains were collected by centrifugation at $3000 \times g$ for 10 min and then washed 3 times with PBS and resuspended with 1 mL of PBS. The cells were lysed using an ultrasonic cell disrupter (Scientz, Beijing, China) and centrifuged at $13,000 \times g$ for 10 min to obtain the supernatant. Then, the supernatant was derivatized with an AccQ·TagTM Chemistry Kit. Finally, the arginine and lysine were analyzed according to our previously established method [27].

2.11. Antimicrobial Susceptibility Testing

Antimicrobial susceptibility was tested using the standardized Bauer–Kirby agar disc diffusion method using Mueller–Hinton agar (Oxoid, CM0337, Basingstoke, Hampshire, UK) and following the instructions of the Clinical Laboratory Standards Institute (CLSI, 2015). *E. coli* ATCC 25,922 was used as a positive control. Discs of 6 antibiotics recommended for Enterobacteriaceae were tested, namely, gentamicin (10 mg), ampicillin (50 mg), penicillin (50 mg), tetracycline (30 mg), ciprofloxacin (5 mg) and kanamycin (50 mg) (Bio-Rad Laboratories, Marnes-la-Coquette, France).

2.12. Statistical Analysis

Data were analyzed using SPSS 19.0 (SPSS Inc., Chicago, IL, USA). The significant differences of the results were assessed by Student's unpaired *t*-test and one-way analysis of variance (ANOVA) [28]. A *P* value of 0.05 was considered statistically significant. The data were presented as means ± deviations, and each experiment was performed in three independent replicate trials.

3. Results

3.1. Verification and Growth Characterization of the ompF Mutant

The gene (ESA_02413) homologous to the *ompF* gene is located in the genome of *C. sakazakii* ATCC BAA-894. The gene is highly similar to the protein sequence of the *ompF* gene of *Salmonella enterica* (92%) and *Enterobacter cloacae* (80%). In order to investigate the functions of *ompF* in *C. sakazakii* ATCC BAA-894 pathogenesis, the *ompF* mutant (Δ*ompF*) was constructed by the Lambda-Red recombination technique. The *ompF* gene was replaced by the kanamycin resistance gene in the Δ*ompF* mutant (Figure 1a), which was confirmed by PCR (Figure 1b) and nucleotide sequencing. Then, we measured the growth curves to observe the effect of *ompF* on bacterial growth rate. Compared with the wild strain, the growth rate of the mutant strain did not show much difference, while that of the complement strain was slightly lower than that of the wild type in the first 6 h, but the difference was not significant (Figure 2a). The morphological characteristics of the wild_type, Δ*ompF* and cp*ompF* strains were examined by SEM, and the results showed that the three strains exhibited similar morphologies (Figure 2b). These results indicated that knocking out the *ompF* gene has no effect on the growth and morphology of *C. sakazakii* in LB medium.

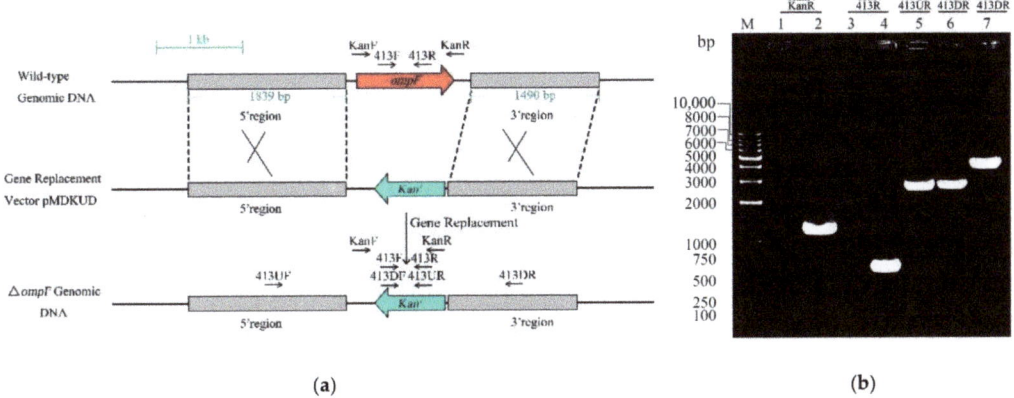

Figure 1. Construction and verification of the *ompF* deletion mutant. (**a**) Schematic representation of the Δ*ompF* construction via homologous recombination. (**b**) Verification of *ompF* homologous recombination events. Lane M, DL10000 marker; lanes 1 and 2, amplified with KF/KR, WT and Δ*ompF* as templates, respectively; lanes 3 and 4, amplified with 413F/413R, Δ*ompF* and WT as templates, respectively; lane 5, amplified with 413UF/413UR, Δ*ompF* as template; lane 6, amplified with 413DF/413DR, Δ*ompF* as template; lane 7, amplified with 413UF/413DR, Δ*ompF* as template.

3.2. Estimation of the Ability to Form Biofilms

A crystal violet staining assay was performed to study the influence of the *ompF* gene on the biofilm formation ability of *C. sakazakii*. Percentages of biofilm formation for the mutant and complementation strains relative to the WT strain are shown in Figure 3. The ability of biofilm formation in Δ*ompF* was significantly less (1.99-fold) than that by WT, while the complement strain showed similar biofilm formation ability to WT. These results indicated that the *ompF* gene played an important role in biofilm formation.

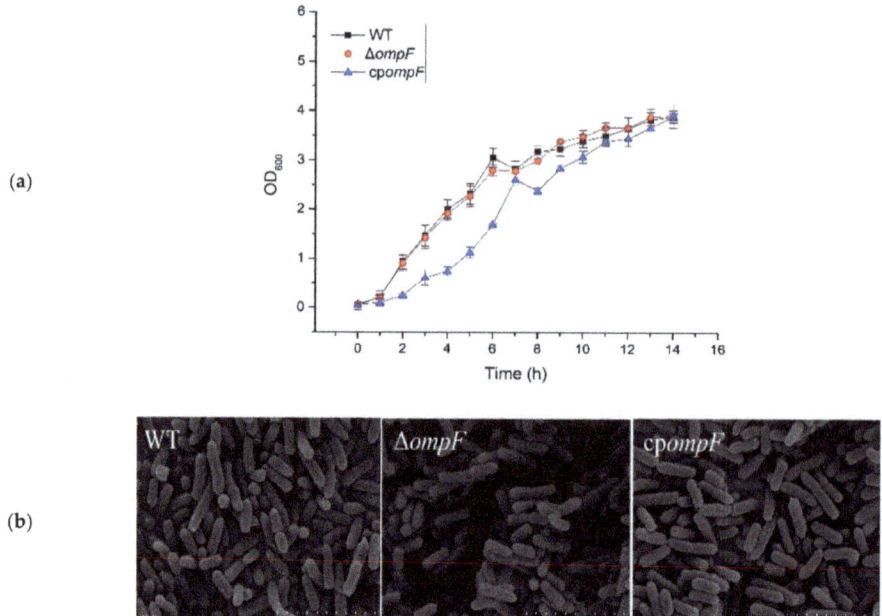

Figure 2. Growth and cell morphology of *C. sakazakii* in LB medium. (**a**) Growth of *C. sakazakii* in LB medium. Error bars represent the standard deviations from independent experiments performed in triplicate. (**b**) SEM to observe the cell morphology of WT, Δ*ompF* and cp*ompF*. Panels: WT, *C. sakazakii* ATCC BAA-894; Δ*ompF*, mutant strain; cp*ompF*, complementation strain.

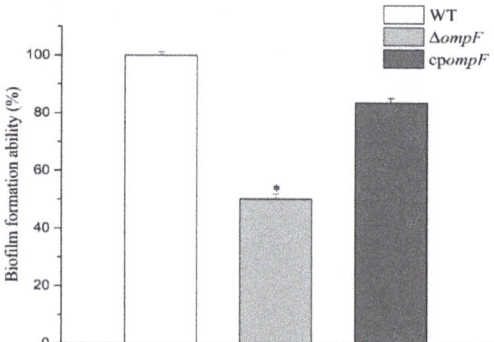

Figure 3. Comparison of the biofilm formation ability of different *C. sakazakii* isolates. The asterisks indicate that the percent biofilm formation by the mutant was significantly different ($p < 0.05$) from that by the wild_type strain.

3.3. Differences in Biofilm Composition Examined by Raman Spectroscopy

In order to explore which components of the biofilm changed after the *ompF* knockout, Raman spectroscopy was performed to further analyze the composition of the *C. sakazakii* biofilm. Additionally, the difference between biofilms formed by WT, Δ*ompF* and cp*ompF* was differentiated by constructing a two-dimensional principal component analysis (PCA) model. There were distinct differences among the Raman peaks representing the biofilm component by the wild_type, mutant and complementation strains (Figure 4a), suggesting that the biochemical components of the three strains are significantly different.

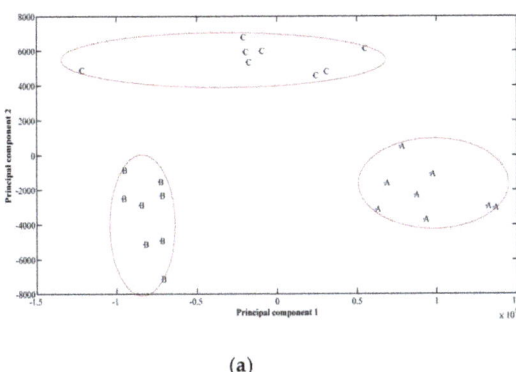 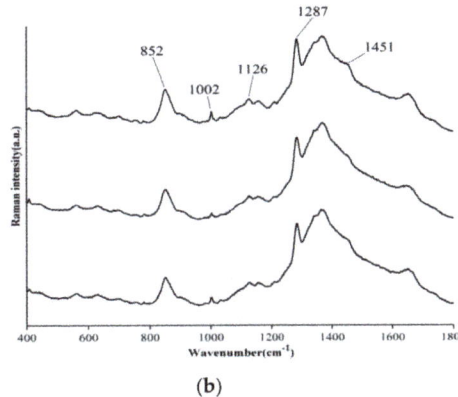

Figure 4. Comparison of the spectral features of *C. sakazakii* biofilms using Raman spectroscopy. (**a**) Principal component analysis of biofilm composition in *C. sakazakii* WT, ΔompF and cpompF strains. (**b**) Comparison of the spectral features of *C. sakazakii* biofilms using Raman spectroscopy. (A): complement strains, (B): mutant, (C): wild_type.

Raman spectra were plotted using MATLAB. A comparison of the Raman spectra suggested that the bands at 852, 1002, 1126, 1287 and 1451 cm^{-1} in ΔompF were lower than those in the WT strain (Figure 4b). Peak assignment was carried out according to previously reported methods [29]. The band characteristic for the common bacterial polysaccharide-(1→3),(1→6)-α-d-glucan is located in 840–60 cm^{-1}, and the bands at 852 cm^{-1} reflected glycogen [30,31]. Spectra of saccharides are characterized by groups of bands in the regions 1000–1200 cm^{-1} and 1002 cm^{-1} reflected β-D-glucose [32], respectively. The band at a wave number of 1126 cm^{-1} was from the skeletal υ(C-C) of the acyl backbones in lipid and disaccharides [30]. The 1287 cm^{-1} band was assigned to the characteristics of phosphodiester groups in nucleic acids, and the 1451 cm^{-1} band reflected fucose and galactosamine [30,32]. These results indicated that the absence of *ompF* negatively affects the content of some saccharides and lipids in biofilms.

3.4. Analysis of the LPS Content of the ompF Mutant and WT Strains

Silver-stained LPS samples isolated from *C. sakazakii* ATCC BAA-894 wild_type, ΔompF and cpompF were analyzed by SDS-PAGE. The LPS profile of ΔompF, including lipid A-core and O-antigen, had a lower molecular weight in contrast to that of the wild type, while the LPS profile of the complement strain was similar to that of WT (Figure 5). From the results, we concluded that *ompF* positively affects the LPS content in *C. sakazakii*.

3.5. ompF Affects Adhesion/Invasion

The ability of adhesion to and invasion of tissue cells is considered to be essential in most pathogenic bacteria. An adhesion/invasion assay was conducted to determine the virulence-related functions of the *ompF* gene in *C. sakazakii*. The ΔompF mutant showed significantly decreased (2.7-fold less than that of the WT) adhesion to and invasion of HCT-8 cells (Figure 6). However, the invasion of HCT-8 cells by the complement strain was similar to that by WT (Figure 6). The results suggested that *ompF* is a positive factor in the process of adhesion to and invasion of host cells by *C. sakazakii*.

3.6. Evaluation of Cell Permeability

As OmpF is a major outer membrane porin that controls the nonspecific diffusion of hydrophilic solutes in *C. sakazakii*, the permeability of the cell membranes of the *C. sakazakii* ATCC BAA-894 wild_type, ΔompF and cpompF was analyzed by measuring the concentration of arginine and lysine. As shown in Table 1, the arginine and lysine concentration of ΔompF was significantly lower than that of the WT. Arginine was not detected in ΔompF, and the concentrations observed in the complement strain were similar to those seen in the

WT strain, indicating that the deletion of *ompF* substantially decreased the permeability of the cell membranes in *C. sakazakii*.

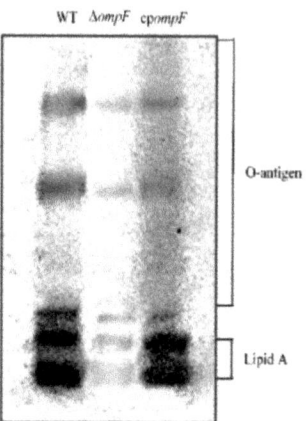

Figure 5. SDS-PAGE analysis of LPS extracted from *C. sakazakii* WT, Δ*ompF* and c*pompF* strains.

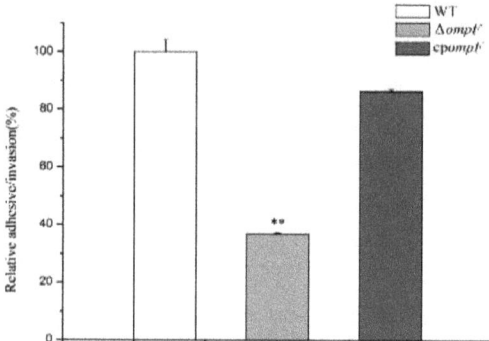

Figure 6. Adhesion to or invasion of epithelial cells by different *C. sakazakii* isolates. The asterisks indicate that the percent invasion by the mutant was significantly different ($p < 0.01$) from that by the wild_type strain.

Table 1. The concentration of arginine and lysine in cell lysates.

Samples	Arginine (μmol·mL^{-1})	Lysine (μmol·mL^{-1})
WT	0.12 ± 0.01 [a]	0.27 ± 0.04 [a]
Δ*ompF*	BDL	0.11 ± 0.03 [b]
c*pompF*	0.09 ± 0.03 [a]	0.27 ± 0.02 [a]

[a,b] Means with different superscript letters within same column are significant different ($p < 0.05$). Values are the means of triplicate samples ± SD. BDL = below detection limit.

3.7. Estimation of Antibiotic Resistance

In order to study the role of the *ompF* gene in the antibiotic resistance of *C. sakazakii*, antimicrobial susceptibility testing was carried out. Based on the size of the inhibition zone, we studied the resistance of the WT, Δ*ompF* and c*pompF* to five small-molecule antibiotics (gentamicin, ampicillin, penicillin, tetracycline and ciprofloxacin). For all four antibiotics, the mutant showed significantly smaller inhibition zones compared to the WT, and the inhibition zones of the complementation strain were similar to those of the WT strain (Figure 7, Table 2). These results suggested that the *ompF* gene encodes a negative effector of antibiotic resistance.

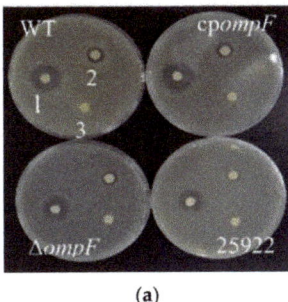
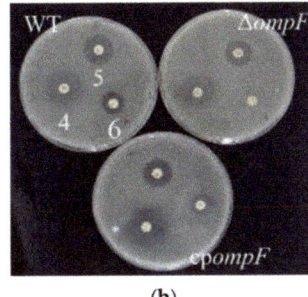

Figure 7. Antibiotic resistance of the *C. sakazakii* WT, ΔompF and cpompF strains. (**a**) 1, 2, 3 and the corresponding positions on the other plates represent gentamicin, ampicillin and penicillin, respectively; (**b**) 4, 5, 6 and the corresponding positions on the other plates represent tetracycline, ciprofloxacin and kanamycin, respectively.

Table 2. Different antibiotic resistance of *C. sakazakii* WT, ΔompF and cpompF strains from the size of inhibition zone.

Antibiotics	Inhibition Zone (mm)			
	WT	ΔompF	cpompF	25922
gentamicin	19.2 ± 0.3 [a]	16.2 ± 0.3 [b]	18.7 ± 0.3 [a]	15.3
amoxicillin	19.7 ± 0.4 [a]	17.6 ± 0.4 [b]	19.7 ± 0.4 [a]	17.4
kanamycin	14.7 ± 0.2 [a]	0.0	14.7 ± 0.3 [a]	17.5
chloramphenicol	19.3 ± 0.9 [a]	17.8 ± 0.5 [b]	18.3 ± 0.4 [a]	-
tetracycline	17.2 ± 0.8 [a]	15.1 ± 0.3 [b]	16.4 ± 0.4 [a]	-
ciprofloxacin	24.6 ± 0.3 [a]	21.5 ± 0.3 [b]	22.4 ± 0.9 [a]	-

[a,b] Means with different superscript letters within same row are significantly different ($p < 0.05$). Values are the means of triplicate samples ± SD.

4. Discussion

Biofilms composed of various major biological macromolecules are aggregates of microorganisms which act as a defense barrier and an important adhesive foundation in biofilm cells [33,34]. In our study, we found that the ability of biofilm formation decreased significantly in the *ompF*-deleted strain, suggesting the involvement of the *ompF* gene in biofilm formation. In addition, the content of some saccharides (glycogen, glucosamine, fucose and galactosamine) and lipids (lipid and phosphodiester groups in nucleic acids) that are constituents of LPS was dramatically higher in WT than that in ΔompF, demonstrating that *ompF* is positively associated with LPS biosynthesis or the binding of LPS to bacterial surfaces. As an important component of biofilms, LPS has been found to play a vital role in biofilm formation in many Gram-negative bacteria [35–37]. In *Actinobacillus pleuropneumoniae* (*A. pleuropneumoniae*), the absence of the LPS O-antigen leads to a decrease in biofilm formation [38]. LPS is an amphipathic molecule that consists of hydrophobic lipid A, inner and outer oligosaccharide cores and O-antigen-specific polysaccharides [39]. The inner core region of LPS is important for outer membrane stability [40]. In *Escherichia coli* K-12, the major pore protein, OmpF, which is assembled as a trimer in the membrane, is tightly bound to the lipopolysaccharide [41]. In addition, Rouslan et al. have reported that the geometry and electrostatics of the OmpF surface make this protein a suitable binding site for LPS in *E. coli* [42]. Consistent with this finding, we speculate that the absence of OmpF in the *ompF* mutant of *C. sakazakii* renders LPS unable to adhere well to the outer membrane. This hypothesis was further confirmed by the SDS-PAGE analysis in this study. We compared the LPS content of the *C. sakazakii* WT and ΔompF strains by SDS-PAGE and observed that the LPS content in the wild_type strain was dramatically higher than that in ΔompF. According to our results, deletion of *ompF* affects the binding of LPS, the main component of biofilms, to the cell membrane, thereby weakening the ability of *C. sakazakii* to form biofilms.

Acting as a defense barrier and an important adhesive foundation in biofilm cells, biofilms are generally defined as an assemblage of microbial cells that adhere to a zoetic or abiotic surface to protect embedded cells against detachment due to flow shear [43]. Many studies have demonstrated that biofilms play an important role in the adherence to and invasion of human epithelial cells by pathogenic bacteria. Byrd et al. found that the biofilm polysaccharide Psl, as an adhesion-associated molecule, is required for adhesion of the bacteria to A549 epithelial cells [44]. In addition, Kunyanee et al. have reported the role of biofilm in the initial attachment and invasion of biofilm-related phenotypes of *B. pseudomallei* in the cellular pathogenesis of human lung epithelial cells [45]. Based on the result that the *C. sakazakii ompF* mutant showed a decreased biofilm formation phenotype, we hypothesized that this gene might be associated with the pathogenicity of *C. sakazakii*. This hypothesis was confirmed by the adhesion/invasion assay. Compared to the parent strain, the ability to adhere to and invade HCT-8 cells was dramatically decreased in the mutant, indicating that *ompF* may be a positive factor in the adhesion to and invasion of tissue cells by *C. sakazakii*. Therefore, *ompF* may regulate adhesion/invasion by affecting biofilm synthesis.

OmpF is one of the most important outer membrane proteins, which provide selective permeability, allowing nutrient molecules and metabolites to enter the cell [46]. It has also been reported that OmpF plays essential roles in the acid resistance of *E. coli* in the presence of arginine and lysine [47]. Therefore, we hypothesized that OmpF contributes to a certain extent to the influx of arginine and lysine across the cell envelope. The HPLC assay showed that the concentration of arginine and lysine in the wild_type strain was significantly greater than that in mutant strains, which directly proved that OmpF has a positive effect on cell permeability in *C. sakazakii*.

OmpF also plays a significant role in the drug resistance of bacteria and has been shown to interact with antibiotics such as β-lactams [48], chloramphenicol [49] and quinolone [50]. In addition, the passage of tetracycline in the magnesium-bound form across the outer membrane appeared to occur preferentially via the porin OmpF [51]. Thus, when OmpF expression decreases, it becomes more difficult for drugs such as tetracyclines, quinolones and β-lactams to enter bacteria [52]. Accordingly, it has been reported that these drugs (ciprofloxacin, trimethoprim, β-lactams, quinolone, etc.) can be used to select for multidrug-resistant mutants that exhibit decreased expression of *ompF* [53,54]. In this study, the resistance to gentamicin, ampicillin, tetracycline and ciprofloxacin of the *ompF* mutant was higher than that of WT, indicating that OmpF plays a vital role in regulating the passage of these antibiotics into *C. sakazakii*.

Interestingly, in the *ompF* complementation strain, some functions were restored; however, the level of *ompF* expression in c*ompF* barely reached those of WT. We propose that such a result may be because the backbone pACYC184 used in c*ompF* belongs to a low-copy-number plasmid. This phenomenon has been reported in our previous study [23]. In addition, Kim et al. reported that the expression level of the *hfq* strain cannot be filled in the *hfq* complement strain prepared using the low-copy-number pACYC184 plasmid in *Cronobacter sakazakii* ATCC 29544. Additionally, the reason may be due to the pACYC184 plasmid harboring *hfq* under a leaky inducible promoter, leading to an imbalance in Hfq production [55].

In our study, the functions of the *ompF* gene were investigated by the gene knockout technique in *C. sakazakii*. We found that this gene played a positive regulatory role in the biofilm formation, and the process is possibly mediated by LPS binding. When the *ompF* gene was knocked out, the content of LPS in the biofilm was significantly reduced in *C. sakazakii*. Furthermore, the results also showed a positive role for *ompF* in the permeability of this bacterium. This study helps to better understand the function of the *ompF* gene in *C. sakazakii* and provides a useful reference for further study of the function of the *ompF* gene in other bacteria.

Supplementary Materials: The following are available online at https://www.mdpi.com/article/10.3390/microorganisms9112338/s1, Table S1: Bacterial strains and plasmids used in this study, Table S2. Primers used in this study, Table S3. Raman intensities of different wavenumbers.

Author Contributions: Conceptualization, J.G., X.D. and S.W.; methodology, J.G. and Z.H.; validation, J.G.; formal analysis, H.Z.; investigation, J.G.; resources, X.D. and S.W.; data curation, P.L.; writing—original draft preparation, J.G.; writing—review and editing, Z.H.; visualization, J.G.; supervision, X.D.; project administration, X.D.; funding acquisition, X.D. and S.W. All authors have read and agreed to the published version of the manuscript.

Funding: This research was funded by The National Science Foundation Project of China, grant number 31972167.

Institutional Review Board Statement: Not applicable.

Informed Consent Statement: Not applicable.

Conflicts of Interest: The authors declare no conflict of interest.

References

1. Blackwood, B.P.; Hunter, C.J. Cronobacter Spp. *Microbiol. Spectr.* **2016**, *4*, 255. [CrossRef]
2. Jin, T.; Guan, N.; Du, Y.; Zhang, X.; Li, J.; Xia, X. *Cronobacter sakazakii* ATCC 29544 translocated human brain microvascular endothelial cells via endocytosis, apoptosis Induction, and disruption of tight junction. *Front. Microbiol.* **2021**, *12*, 675020. [CrossRef]
3. Forsythe, S.J.; Dickins, B.; Jolley, K.A. *Cronobacter*, the emergent bacterial pathogen *Enterobacter sakazakii* comes of age; MLST and whole genome sequence analysis. *BMC Genom.* **2014**, *15*, 1121. [CrossRef]
4. Joseph, S.; Desai, P.; Ji, Y.; Cummings, C.A.; Shih, R.; Degoricija, L.; Rico, A.; Brzoska, P.; Hamby, S.E.; Masood, N.; et al. Comparative analysis of genome sequences covering the seven *Cronobacter* species. *PLoS ONE* **2012**, *7*, e49455. [CrossRef] [PubMed]
5. Morato Rodríguez, M.D.; Velandia Rodríguez, D.; Castañeda, S.; Crosby, M.; Vera, H. *Cronobacter spp.* in Common Breast Milk Substitutes, Bogotá, Colombia. *Emerg. Infect. Dis.* **2018**, *24*, 1907–1909. [CrossRef]
6. Ling, N.; Jiang, Y.; Zeng, H.; Ding, Y.; Forsythe, S. Advances in our understanding and distribution of the *Cronobacter* genus in China. *Int. J. Food Microbiol. J. Food Sci.* **2021**, *86*, 276–283.
7. Marotta, S.M.; Giarratana, F.; Calvagna, A.; Ziino, G.; Giuffrida, A.; Panebianco, A. Study on microbial communities in domestic kitchen sponges: Evidence of *Cronobacter sakazakii* and Extended Spectrum Beta Lactamase (ESBL) producing bacteria. *Ital. J. Food Saf.* **2018**, *7*, 7672. [CrossRef]
8. Almajed, F.S.; Forsythe, S.J. *Cronobacter sakazakii* clinical isolates overcome host barriers and evade the immune response. *Microb. Pathog.* **2016**, *90*, 55–63. [CrossRef] [PubMed]
9. Furukawa, S.; Kuchma, S.L.; O'Toole, G.A. Keeping their options open: Acute versus persistent infections. *J. Bacteriol.* **2006**, *188*, 1211–1217. [CrossRef]
10. Lehner, A.; Riedel, K.; Eberl, L.; Breeuwer, P.; Diep, B.; Stephan, R. Biofilm formation, extracellular polysaccharide production, and cell-to-cell signaling in various *Enterobacter sakazakii* strains: Aspects promoting environmental persistence. *J. Food Prot.* **2005**, *68*, 2287–2294. [CrossRef] [PubMed]
11. Kim, H.; Ryu, J.H.; Beuchat, L.R. Attachment of and biofilm formation by *Enterobacter sakazakii* on stainless steel and enteral feeding tubes. *Appl. Environ. Microbiol.* **2006**, *72*, 5846–5856. [CrossRef] [PubMed]
12. Hartmann, I.; Carranza, P.; Lehner, A.; Stephan, R.; Eberl, L.; Riedel, K. Genes involved in *Cronobacter sakazakii* biofilm formation. *Appl. Environ. Microbiol.* **2010**, *76*, 2251–2261. [CrossRef] [PubMed]
13. Achouak, W.; Heulin, T.; Pagès, J.M. Multiple facets of bacterial porins. *FEMS Microbiol. Lett.* **2001**, *199*, 1–7. [CrossRef]
14. Hatfaludi, T.; Al-Hasani, K.; Boyce, J.D.; Adler, B. Outer membrane proteins of Pasteurella multocida. *Vet. Microbiol.* **2010**, *144*, 1–17. [CrossRef] [PubMed]
15. Im, W.; Roux, B. Ion permeation and selectivity of OmpF porin: A theoretical study based on molecular dynamics, brownian dynamics, and continuum electrodiffusion theory. *J. Mol. Biol.* **2002**, *322*, 851–869. [CrossRef]
16. Varma, S.; Chiu, S.W.; Jakobsson, E. The influence of amino acid protonation states on molecular dynamics simulations of the bacterial porin OmpF. *Biophys. J.* **2006**, *90*, 112–123. [CrossRef]
17. Prehna, G.; Zhang, G.; Gong, X.; Duszyk, M.; Okon, M.; McIntosh, L.P.; Weiner, J.H.; Strynadka, N.C. A protein export pathway involving *Escherichia coli* porins. *Structure* **2012**, *20*, 1154–1166. [CrossRef]
18. Nestorovich, E.M.; Rostovtseva, T.K.; Bezrukov, S.M. Residue ionization and ion transport through OmpF channels. *Biophys. J.* **2003**, *85*, 3718–3729. [CrossRef]
19. Kojima, S.; Nikaido, H. Permeation rates of penicillins indicate that *Escherichia coli* porins function principally as nonspecific channels. *Proc. Natl. Acad. Sci. USA* **2013**, *110*, 2629–2634. [CrossRef]

20. Kim, K.; Kim, K.P.; Choi, J.; Lim, J.A.; Lee, J.; Hwang, S.; Ryu, S. Outer membrane proteins A (OmpA) and X (OmpX) are essential for basolateral invasion of *Cronobacter sakazakii*. *Appl. Environ. Microbiol.* **2010**, *76*, 5188–5198. [CrossRef]
21. Chang, A.C.; Cohen, S.N. Construction and characterization of amplifiable multicopy DNA cloning vehicles derived from the P15A cryptic miniplasmid. *J. Bacteriol.* **1978**, *134*, 1141–1156. [CrossRef]
22. Hu, L.; Grim, C.J.; Franco, A.A.; Jarvis, K.G.; Sathyamoorthy, V.; Kothary, M.H.; McCardell, B.A.; Tall, B.D. Analysis of the cellulose synthase operon genes, bcsA, bcsB, and bcsC in Cronobacter species: Prevalence among species and their roles in biofilm formation and cellcell aggregation. *Food Microbiol.* **2015**, *52*, 97–105. [CrossRef] [PubMed]
23. Gao, J.X.; Li, P.; Du, X.J.; Han, Z.H.; Xue, R.; Liang, B.; Wang, S. A Negative Regulator of Cellulose Biosynthesis, bcsR, Affects Biofilm Formation, and Adhesion/Invasion Ability of *Cronobacter sakazakii*. *Front. Microbiol.* **2017**, *8*, 1839. [CrossRef]
24. Hong, T.P.; Carter, M.Q.; Struffi, P.; Casonato, S.; Hao, Y.; Lam, J.S.; Lory, S.; Jousson, O. Conjugative type IVb pilus recognizes lipopolysaccharide of recipient cells to initiate PAPI-1 pathogenicity island transfer in *Pseudomonas aeruginosa*. *BMC Microbiol.* **2017**, *17*, 31. [CrossRef] [PubMed]
25. Yan, Q.; Jarvis, K.G.; Chase, H.R.; Hebert, K.; Trach, L.H.; Lee, C.; Sadowski, J.; Lee, B.; Hwang, S.; Sathyamoorthy, V.; et al. A proposed harmonized LPS molecular-subtyping scheme for *Cronobacter* species. *Food Microbiol.* **2015**, *50*, 38–43. [CrossRef]
26. Rogers, T.J.; Thorpe, C.M.; Paton, A.W.; Paton, J.C. Role of lipid rafts and flagellin in invasion of colonic epithelial cells by Shiga-Toxigenic *Escherichia coli* O113:H21. *Infect. Immun.* **2012**, *80*, 2858–2867. [CrossRef]
27. Han, Z.H.; Liu, B.; Niu, Z.Y.; Zhang, Y.; Gao, J.X.; Shi, L.; Wang, S.J.; Wang, S. Role of α-Dicarbonyl Compounds in the Inhibition Effect of Reducing Sugars on the Formation of 2-Amino-1-methyl-6-phenylimidazo[4,5-b]pyridine. *J. Agric. Food Chem.* **2017**, *65*, 10084–10092. [CrossRef] [PubMed]
28. Mccullagh, P. Discussion of "Analysis of variance-why it is more important than ever" by A. Gelman. *Ann. Stat.* **2005**, *33*, 34–40.
29. Du, X.J.; Zhang, X.; Li, P.; Xue, R.; Wang, S. Screening of genes involved in interactions with intestinal epithelial cells in *Cronobacter sakazakii*. *AMB Express* **2016**, *6*, 74. [CrossRef] [PubMed]
30. Movasaghi, Z.; Rehman, S.; Rehman, I.U. Raman spectroscopy of biological tissues. *Appl. Spectrosc. Rev.* **2007**, *42*, 493–541. [CrossRef]
31. Gelder, J.D.; Gussem, K.D.; Vandenabeele, P.; Moens, L. Reference database of Raman spectra of biological molecules. *J. Raman Spectrosc.* **2007**, *38*, 1133–1147. [CrossRef]
32. Gieroba, B.; Krysa, M.; Wojtowicz, K.; Wiater, A.; Pleszczy'nska, M.; Tomczyk, M.; Sroka-Bartnicka, A. The FT-IR and Raman Spectroscopies as Tools for Biofilm Characterization Created by Cariogenic Streptococci. *Int. J. Mol. Sci.* **2020**, *21*, 3811. [CrossRef]
33. Serra, D.O.; Richter, A.M.; Hengge, R. Cellulose as an architectural element in spatially structured *Escherichia coli* biofilms. *J. Bacteriol.* **2013**, *195*, 5540–5554. [CrossRef] [PubMed]
34. Kolter, R.; Greenberg, E.P. Microbial sciences-The superficial life of microbes. *Nature* **2006**, *441*, 300–302. [CrossRef]
35. Puttamreddy, S.; Cornick, N.A.; Minion, F.C. Genome-wide transposon mutagenesis reveals a role for pO157 genes in biofilm development in *Escherichia coli* O157:H7 EDL933. *Infect. Immun.* **2010**, *78*, 2377–2384. [CrossRef]
36. De Araujo, C.; Balestrino, D.; Roth, L.; Charbonnel, N.; Forestier, C. Quorum sensing affects biofilm formation through lipopolysaccharide synthesis in *Klebsiella pneumoniae*. *Res. Microbiol.* **2010**, *161*, 595–603. [CrossRef] [PubMed]
37. Lau, P.C.; Lindhout, T.; Beveridge, T.J.; Dutcher, J.R.; Lam, J.S. Differential lipopolysaccharide core capping leads to quantitative and correlated modifications of mechanical and structural properties in *Pseudomonas aeruginosa* biofilms. *J. Bacteriol.* **2009**, *191*, 6618–6631. [CrossRef]
38. Hathroubi, S.; Hancock, M.A.; Bosse, J.T.; Langford, P.R.; Tremblay, Y.D.; Labrie, J.; Jacques, M. Surface polysaccharide mutants reveal that absence of O antigen reduces biofilm formation of *Actinobacillus pleuropneumoniae*. *Infect. Immun.* **2016**, *84*, 127–137. [CrossRef] [PubMed]
39. Wang, X.; Quinn, P.J. Lipopolysaccharide: Biosynthetic pathway and structure modification. *Prog. Lipid Res.* **2010**, *49*, 97–107. [CrossRef]
40. Brabetz, W.; Muller-Loennies, S.; Holst, O.; Brade, H. Deletion of the heptosyltransferase genes rfaC and rfaF in *Escherichia coli* K-12 results in a Re-type lipopolysaccharide with a high degree of 2-aminoethanol phosphate substitution. *Eur. J. Biochem.* **1997**, *247*, 716–724. [CrossRef] [PubMed]
41. Fourel, D.; Mizushima, S.; Bernadac, A.; Pagès, J.M. Specific regions of *Escherichia coli* OmpF protein involved in antigenic and colicin receptor sites and in stable trimerization. *J. Bacteriol.* **1993**, *175*, 2754–2757. [CrossRef]
42. Efremov, R.G.; Sazanov, L.A. Structure of Escherichia coli OmpF porin from lipidic mesophase. *J. Struct. Biol.* **2012**, *178*, 311–318. [CrossRef] [PubMed]
43. Aparna, M.S.; Yadav, S. Biofilms: Microbes and disease. *Braz. J. Infect. Dis.* **2008**, *12*, 526–530. [CrossRef] [PubMed]
44. Byrd, M.S.; Pang, B.; Mishra, M.; Swords, W.E.; Wozniak, D.J. The *Pseudomonas aeruginosa* exopolysaccharide Psl facilitates surface adherence and NF-kappa B activation in A549 cells. *mBio* **2010**, *1*, e00140-10. [CrossRef] [PubMed]
45. Kunyanee, C.; Kamjumphol, W.; Taweechaisupapong, S.; Kanthawong, S.; Wongwajana, S.; Wongratanacheewin, S.; Hahnvajanawong, C.; Chareonsudjai, S. Burkholderia pseudomallei biofilm promotes adhesion, internalization and stimulates proinflammatory cytokines in human epithelial A549 Cells. *PLoS ONE* **2016**, *11*, e0160741. [CrossRef] [PubMed]
46. Jap, B.K.; Walian, P.J. Structure and functional mechanism of porins. *Physiol. Rev.* **1996**, *76*, 1073–1088. [CrossRef] [PubMed]
47. Bekhit, A.; Fukamachi, T.; Saito, H.; Kobayashi, H. The role of OmpC and OmpF in acidic resistance in *Escherichia Coli*. *Biol. Pharm. Bull.* **2011**, *34*, 330–334. [CrossRef]

48. Jeanteur, D.; Schirmer, T.; Fourel, D.; Simonet, V.; Rummel, G.; Widmer, C.; Pages, J.M. Structural and functional alterations of a colicin-resistant mutant of OmpF porin from *Escherichia Coli*. *Proc. Natl. Acad. Sci. USA* **1994**, *91*, 10675–10679. [CrossRef]
49. Jaktaji, R.P.; Ebadi, R. Study the expression of marA gene in ciprofloxacin and tetracycline resistant mutants of *Esherichia Coli*. *Iran J. Pharm. Res.* **2013**, *12*, 923–928.
50. Law, C.J.; Penfold, C.N.; Walker, D.C.; Moore, G.R.; James, R.; Kleanthous, C. OmpF enhances the ability of BtuB to protect susceptible *Escherichia coli* cells from colicin E9 cytotoxicity. *FEBS Lett.* **2003**, *545*, 127–132. [CrossRef]
51. Thanassi, D.G.; Suh, G.S.; Nikaido, H. Role of outer membrane barrier in efflux-mediated tetracycline resistance of *Escherichia Coli*. *J. Bacterial.* **1995**, *177*, 998–1007. [CrossRef] [PubMed]
52. Kishii, R.; Takei, M. Relationship between the expression of *ompF* and quinolone resistance in *Escherichia Coli*. *J. Infect. Chemother.* **2009**, *15*, 361–366. [CrossRef]
53. Tavío, M.M.; Vila, J.; Ruiz, J.; Ruiz, J.; Martín-Sánchez, A.M.; Jiménez de Anta, M.T. Mechanisms involved in the development of resistance to fluoroquinolones in *Escherichia coli* isolates. *J. Antimicrob. Chemother.* **1999**, *44*, 735–742. [CrossRef] [PubMed]
54. Miller, K.; O'Neill, A.J.; Chopra, I. *Escherichia coli* mutators present an enhanced risk for emergence of antibiotic resistance during urinary tract infections. *Antimicrob. Agents Chemother.* **2004**, *48*, 23–29. [CrossRef]
55. Kim, S.; Hwang, H.; Kim, K.P.; Yoon, H.; Kang, D.H.; Ryu, S. *hfq* Plays important roles in virulence and stress adaptation in *Cronobacter sakazakii* ATCC 29544. *Infect. Immun.* **2015**, *83*, 2089–2098. [CrossRef] [PubMed]

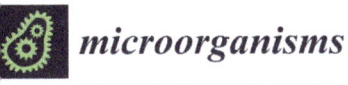

Article

K1 Antigen Is Associated with Different AST Profile in *Escherichia coli*: A One-Month-Long Pilot Study

Maelys Proquot [1], Lovasoa Najaraly Jamal [1], Chloe Plouzeau-Jayle [1], Anthony Michaud [1], Lauranne Broutin [1], Christophe Burucoa [1,2], Julie Cremniter [1,2] and Maxime Pichon [1,2,*]

[1] Bacteriology and Infection Control Laboratory, Infectious Agents Department, University Hospital of Poitiers, 86021 Poitiers, France; maelys.proquot@etu.univ-poitiers.fr (M.P.); lovasoa.najaraly.jamal@etu.univ-poitiers.fr (L.N.J.); chloe.plouzeau-jayle@chu-poitiers.fr (C.P.-J.); anthony.michaud@chu-poitiers.fr (A.M.); lauranne.broutin@chu-poitiers.fr (L.B.); christophe.burucoa@chu-poitiers.fr (C.B.); julie.cremniter@chu-poitiers.fr (J.C.)

[2] INSERM U1070 Pharmacology of Antimicrobial Agents, Faculty of Medicine and Pharmacy, University of Poitiers, 86021 Poitiers, France

* Correspondence: maxime.pichon@chu-poitiers.fr; Tel.: +33-(0)-549-444-143

Abstract: *Escherichia coli* is responsible for diseases of varying severity. The "K" antigen designates the capsular polysaccharides on the bacterial surface, which are mostly similar to those of highly pathogenic bacteria. The K1 antigen is often found in pathogenic *E. coli*. Aim: While the published studies on the AST profile of K1-positive *E. coli* have focused on pregnant women or newborns, this study aimed to characterize the AST profile of K1-positive *E. coli* independently of the clinical sample of isolation. Over a 4-week-long period, all patients hospitalized/consulting at the Poitiers University Hospital presenting a determined AST on *E. coli* were prospectively included to define their K1-status (Pastorex Meningitis) and to collect the clinical (age/sex) or biological metadata (AST/MIC). Among the 296 included samples, no differential representation was observed between K1 results regarding sample nature. K1-negative results were associated with multiple antibiotic-resistance (12.3% vs. 33.0%; $p < 0.01$). AST phenotypes differed between these groups, with a higher proportion of K1-negativity among resistant strains, especially on β-lactams (ureidopenicillin, 25.8% vs. 14.9%; and ampicillin/inhibitor, 50.0% vs. 26.8%; $p < 0.05$) or quinolone (19.8% vs. 7.0%) and sulfamethoxazole-trimethoprim (30.2% vs. 12.3%) ($p < 0.01$). This study analyzed *E. coli* ASTs in clinical samples of all types, regarding their K1-antigen status.

Keywords: *Escherichia coli*; K1 antigen; virulence; maternal-fetal infection; antibiotic susceptibility testing; resistance to antimicrobial agents

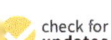

Citation: Proquot, M.; Jamal, L.N.; Plouzeau-Jayle, C.; Michaud, A.; Broutin, L.; Burucoa, C.; Cremniter, J.; Pichon, M. K1 Antigen Is Associated with Different AST Profile in *Escherichia coli*: A One-Month-Long Pilot Study. *Microorganisms* **2021**, *9*, 884. https://doi.org/10.3390/microorganisms9091884

Academic Editors: Dobroslava Bujňáková, Nikola Puvača and Ivana Ćirković

Received: 20 July 2021
Accepted: 31 August 2021
Published: 5 September 2021

Publisher's Note: MDPI stays neutral with regard to jurisdictional claims in published maps and institutional affiliations.

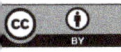

Copyright: © 2021 by the authors. Licensee MDPI, Basel, Switzerland. This article is an open access article distributed under the terms and conditions of the Creative Commons Attribution (CC BY) license (https://creativecommons.org/licenses/by/4.0/).

1. Introduction

Escherichia coli is physiologically a normal inhabitant of the gastrointestinal tract of healthy humans. Under particular conditions, this bacterium may localize in various tissues and be responsible for very diverse diseases [1]. The term K antigen was introduced by Kauffmann et al. to designate a surface structure [2]. To date, most of the categorized K antigens are capsular polysaccharides, similar in their overall properties to the capsular saccharides of highly pathogenic and invasive bacteria, such as *Neisseria meningitidis*, *Streptococcus pneumoniae* or *Haemophilus influenzae* [3–5]. Among virulence factors that enable these bacteria to survive and to grow in its host, K1 capsular polysaccharide is often found in pathogenic *E. coli*. The relation between capsular polysaccharides and invasiveness of *E. coli* was first suggested by Smith and then Kauffman [6,7]. Invasiveness was postulated to be their anticomplementary effect [8,9]. The variability of virulence marker expression influences the characteristics of the bacteria, which can finally lead to different phenotypes and antibiotic susceptibility testing (AST) under laboratory examinations in vitro. Depending on the circumstances, the physiological state of the patient and the virulence factors,

E. coli is one of the main causative agents of both gastrointestinal and non-gastrointestinal infections [10].

Pathogenic E. coli bacteria remain a major source of morbidity and mortality, mainly due to neonatal bacterial meningitis [11]. Some of these diseases can lead to death, and among survivors more than fifty percent present serious neurological conditions (seizure disorders, hydrocephalus, developmental delay and hearing loss). Other clinical diseases are caused by K1 capsular serotype, including urinary tract infection (more than 50%) and bacteremia (approximately ten to fifteen percent of adult E. coli-caused bacteremia originate from K1-positive strains) [12].

Even if these mechanisms have been shown to differ from the ones of group B streptococci and Listeria monocytogenes, K1 capsule antigen is a key virulence factor in the pathogenesis of E. coli meningitis. This factor allows E. coli to internalize itself into human brain microvascular endothelial cells via a mechanism requiring host cell actin cytoskeleton and transduction pathways [13]. This internalization and pathophysiological process implicates other virulence mechanisms, such as P-fimbriae and outer membrane protein A. The latter has often been researched when focusing on virulence characterization of E. coli [14]. Moreover, E. coli K1-positive-containing vacuoles are not fused with lysosomes, thereby allowing E. coli to cross the blood–brain barrier as living bacteria, which not only allows it to resist most of the macrophage properties, but also has a bearing on its serum resistance [13].

As for virulence determinants, the expression of antibiotic resistance in Enterobacteriaceae, such as E. coli, is controlled by different environmental signals [15]. More recently, as the genotypic characterization of E. coli has improved, the impact and need for understanding of non-gastrointestinal strains has become ever more evident. Indeed, these strains represent an increasing problem for human health management, especially due to the major incidence of antibiotic resistance, often carried by plasmid in gram-negative bacteria (accounting for 64% of the bacterial strains identified in Indian neonates presenting extended spectrum beta-lactamase) [16,17]. As concerns maternal-fetal infection, most of the studies published to date have focused on the characteristics of vaginal and/or rectal E. coli of pregnant woman, in association with a particular AST profile. Neonatal E. coli strains have demonstrated resistance to aminopenicillins as high as 100%, 78% and 93% (and 90%, 10% and 28% to aminoglycosides) in developing countries, the USA and Spain respectively [18–21].

While most of the published studies focusing on the AST profile of K1-antigenic E. coli implicated in diseases are focused on pregnant women or newborns and neonates, the present study aimed to characterize the AST profile of K1-antigenic E. coli among all identified strains in analyzed samples in both adults and children.

2. Materials and Methods

2.1. Selection Criteria and Demographic/Clinical Characteristics

All hospitalized or consulting patients at the University Hospital of Poitiers in whom Escherichia coli was identified and tested for AST were prospectively included over a four-week period (18 January to 14 February 2021). In all included patients, the first bacterial strains for which an AST was performed were collected (in the case of two different aspects, both were considered for further analyses, including AST and K1 determination). If E. coli was identified in two different locations/samples on a particular day, the more severe location was preferred (for example: positive blood culture was considered as a reflection of a condition more severe than positive urine culture).

For all included patients, a clinical record file was completed, leading to an anonymized database that included all clinical (age, gender, hospitalization location and type of sampling) or biological metadata (AST results or MIC determination if available, K1 determination when carried out in routine treatment in the usual management of the patient).

2.2. AST Determination

After overnight culture, the susceptibility of *E. coli* strains to antimicrobial agents was analyzed by disc-diffusion (i2a, Montpellier, France) on Muller-Hinton (MH) agar (BioRad, Hercules, CA, USA) (for bacterial strains identified in blood culture) or liquid method on Vitek 2 system (bioMérieux, Marcy-l'étoile, France) (for bacterial strains identified in all samples but blood culture). All analytical processes and threshold determinations were evaluated according to the European Committee on Antimicrobial Susceptibility Testing (CA-SFM/EUCAST—April 2020). For all tested strains, AST was interpreted by a senior medical biologist (C. P-J; A.M.; L.B.; CB; J.C. or M.P), to validate technical results and centralize them in a single database. Following collection of the results, the medical biologist responsible for the study (M.P.) classified the bacterial strains according to their phenotypic mode of resistance.

2.3. K1 Phenotypic Determination

After the overnight growth of MH agar (BioRad), bacterial colonies were isolated and then the K1 antigen-status was determined using the Pastorex Meningitis kits (Bio-Rad, CA, USA) according to the manufacturer's recommendations. Briefly, this test employs latex beads covered by mouse monoclonal antibodies specific to *E. coli* K1. In the presence of the K1 antigen, the latex particles are visually agglutinated when they remain in a homogeneous suspension in the absence of this antigen. Positive control was verified using particles sensitized with the mouse monoclonal antibody specific to *E. coli* K1, and negative control consisted of particles sensitized with IgG immunoglobulins from a non-immunized rabbit.

2.4. Statistical Analyses

Statistical analyses were performed with GraphPad Prism version 9.0. Descriptive statistics were used to analyze both parametric and nonparametric data as appropriate. The Fisher exact test was used to compare proportions. An unpaired t-test was used to compare continuous data after validation of the normality distribution of the data using a Shapiro-Wilk test. A *p*-value below 0.05 was considered as significant and a *p*-value below 0.01 as very significant.

2.5. Ethical Considerations

All the biological and clinical records used in the present study were pseudonymized before analysis. In French laws, explicit consent of the patient is not needed for this type of analyses.

3. Results

3.1. Demographic Characteristics of the Cohort

During the period of inclusion, 296 samples could be selected according to the pre-specified inclusion criteria among the 639 samples (46.3%) diagnosed with *E. coli* at the Bacteriology laboratory of the Infectious Agents Department (CHU de Poitiers, France). This inclusion rate allowed the detection of a difference of 20%, with a confidence interval of 95% and a power of 90%.

Among the tested strains ($n = 296$), 114 were characterized as K1-positive strains (39.9%) and 182 (60.1%) as K1 negative strains.

3.2. K1-Antigen Distribution through Clinical Sample Type

All the clinical and biological characteristics of the included patients are summarized in Table 1. No difference could be observed in terms of sex or age between groups ($p > 0.05$). Samples were mainly urine samples (including less than one fifth of those using catheter) followed by blood culture and genital samples. No difference was observed comparing the time-to-positive culture (17.4 vs. 12.8 h) for blood culture ($p > 0.05$).

Table 1. Demographic characteristics and sample nature of the analyzed cohort.

	Demographic or Biological Parameters	K1-Positive Strain (n = 114)	K1-Negative Strain (n = 182)
	Sex (M/F)	31/83	49/133
	Age (mean, SD)	61.9 (27.3)	61.3 (27.7)
Sample nature (n, % of the whole group)	Urine sample (all) (n = 235, 79.4% of the whole cohort)	90 (38.3)	145 (61.7)
	Urine sample (catheter) (n = 37) (% of the urine sample group)	16 (17.8)	21 (11.5)
	Blood sample (n = 31; 10.5% of the whole cohort)	12 (38.7)	19 (61.3)
	Genital sample (n = 11; 3.7% of the whole cohort)	4 (36.4)	7 (63.6)
	Genital sample (Female) (n = 10) (% of the genital sample group)	3 (75)	7 (100)
	Puncture fluid (n = 11; 3.7% of the whole cohort)	3 (27.3)	8 (72.7)
	Neonatal sample (Gastric lavage, Placenta) (n = 4; 1.4% of the whole cohort)	2 (50)	2 (50)
	Respiratory sample (n = 2; 0.7% of the whole cohort)	2 (100)	0 (0)
	Otolaryngology—Ophthalmology Sample (n = 2; 0.7% of the whole cohort)	1 (50)	1 (50)

3.3. Distribution of AST Phenotypes among K1-Positive and K1-Negative Strains

All AST results were analyzed after the K1-phenotype characterization and during routine biological management of the samples. The profiles are summarized in Table 2.

Table 2. Comparison of the AST phenotypes per antibiotic molecules.

	Antibiotic Susceptibility Testing Results	K1-Positive Strain (n; %)	K1-Negative Strain (n; %)	p-Value
	β lactam (n = 296)			
	All susceptible (n = 123)	53 (46.5)	70 (38.5)	-
	≥1 Resistance (n = 173)	61 (53.5)	112 (61.5)	-
	Ampicillin-resistant (n = 137/296; 46.3%)	45 (39.5)	92 (50.5)	-
	Ticarcillin-resistant (n = 133/296)	42 (26.8)	91 (50.0)	<0.05
	Resistance to Ampicillin + inhibitor (n = 64/296)	17 (14.9)	47 (25.8)	<0.05
	Resistance to Ticarcillin + inhibitor (n = 11/24)	3 (37.5)	8 (50.0)	-
	Resistance to Piperacillin + inhibitor (n = 24/296)	6 (5.3)	18 (9.9)	-
	ESBL (n = 8/296)	2 (1.8)	6 (3.3)	-
	Resistance to 2nd gen. Cephalosporin (n = 9/262)	2 (1.8)	7 (4.7)	-
	Resistance to 3rd gen. Cephalosporin (n = 7/296)	2 (1.8)	5 (2.7)	-
	Resistance to 4th gen. Cephalosporin (n = 2/24)	1 (11.1)	1 (6.7)	-
	Temocillin-resistant (n = 41/258)	16 (16.2)	25 (15.7)	-
	Aztreonam-resistant (n = 3/19)	1 (12.5)	2 (18.2)	-
	Carbapenem-resistant (n = 0/296; 0%)	0 (-)	0 (-)	-
	Aminoglycoside-resistant (n = 11/296)			
	All	2 (1.75)	9 (4.94)	-
	G (n = 8)	2 (100)	6 (66.7)	-
	GT (n = 1)	0 (-)	1 (11.1)	-
	A (n = 2)	0 (-)	2 (22.2)	-
Quinolones (n = 44/296)	All	8 (7.0)	36 (19.8)	<0.01
	Nalidixic acid only (n = 2) (% of the quinolone-resistant subgroup)	0 (0)	2 (100)	-
	Quinolones-resistant (n = 44/296)	8 (7.0)	36 (19.8)	<0.01
	Trimethoprim—sulfamethoxazole -resistant (n = 69/296)	14 (12.3)	55 (30.2)	<0.01
	Furan-resistant (n = 1/275)	0 (-)	1 (0.6)	-
	Fosfomycin-resistant (n = 4/259)	1 (1.0)	3 (1.9)	-

ESBL: extended-spectrum beta-lactamase; G: resistance to Gentamycin only; GT: resistance to Gentamycin and Tobramycin only; A: resistance to Amikacin.

For resistance to β lactam no difference could be observed between groups in prevalence for all susceptible strains, or for ampicillin, ticarcillin/piperacillin associated with beta-lactamase inhibitor, cephalosporin or carbapenem. Few ESBL-bearing *E. coli* were observed in this study without a difference between groups. Differences were observed regarding resistance to the ampicillin with the inhibitor and the ticarcillin, with higher prevalence in K1-negative strains compared to K1-positive strains (50.0% vs. 26.8% and 25.8% vs. 14.9% respectively; $p < 0.05$).

For resistance to quinolone, a higher proportion of resistant strains was observed in K1-negative strains (19.8% vs. 7.0%; $p < 0.01$), without any difference in terms of level of quinolone resistance (nalidixic acid only or associated with other quinolone; $p > 0.05$).

For resistance to Sulfamethoxazole—trimethoprim, a higher proportion of resistant strains was observed in K1-negative strains (30.2% vs. 12.3%; $p < 0.01$). On the contrary, differences could be observed between groups, in terms of resistance to aminoglycosides, furans and Fosfomycin ($p > 0.05$).

3.4. Proportion of Pluri-Resistant Strains According to K1-Antigen Status

After the exploration of antibiotic-resistance per family, antibiotic resistance was explored regarding pluri-resistance status (defined in this study as a strain resistant to at least two different classes among tested ones) (Table 3.). For this purpose, antibiotic molecules were categorized into six different classes (i.e., β lactam, aminoglycosides, quinolones, furanes, fosfomycins and sulfamethoxazoles-trimethoprim). Due to different recommendations for testing, not all classes were tested, and to overcome this possible bias, only β lactam, aminoglycosides, quinolones and sulfamethoxazole-trimethoprim were included for the class-by-class analysis when all classes were considered for numerical determination of pluri-resistance.

Table 3. Comparison of the AST multi-resistant phenotypes.

Antibiotic Susceptibility Testing Results	K1-Positive Strain ($n = 114$)	K1-Negative Strain ($n = 182$)	p-Value
Pluri-resistance (n; %)	21 (18.4)	76 (41.8)	<0.01
Number of antimicrobial classes incompletely susceptible * (mean; SEM)	0.68 (0.07)	1.11 (0.08)	<0.01
Number of strains presenting X incompletely susceptible antimicrobial classes **			
1 class ($n = 104$; 35.1%)	46 (40.4)	58 (31.9)	-
2 classes ($n = 56$; 18.9%)	12 (10.5)	44 (24.2)	<0.01
3 classes ($n = 13$; 4.4%)	2 (1.8)	11 (6.0)	- ***
4 classes ($n = 5$; 1.7%)	0 (0)	5 (2.7)	-

* Classes were: B-lactam; aminoglycosides; Quinolones; Fosfomycin; Trimethoprim—sulfamethoxazole; furans; ** Classes were: B-lactam; aminoglycosides; Quinolones; Trimethoprim—sulfamethoxazole; *** statistical trends (p value < 0.1); SEM: Standard Error of the Mean.

Regarding the number of classes that were incompletely susceptible (or resistant), a difference of proportion was observed for strains with altered susceptibility to at least two antibiotic classes (12.3% vs. 33.0%; $p < 0.01$). This was confirmed by the higher mean number of antimicrobial classes the bacterial strain was resistant to, in K1-negative strains compared to K1-positive ones (0.68 vs. 1.11; $p < 0.01$). This difference tends to decrease for a larger number of classes (13.7% for two classes; 3.2% for three classes and 2.7% for four classes), without statistical difference for strains with altered susceptibility to three out of four classes ($p > 0.05$).

4. Discussion

This study is the first, to the best of our knowledge, to analyze antibiotic resistance of *E. coli* isolated from clinical samples of all types, regarding their K1-antigen status in both hospitalized and ambulatory patients.

The association between virulence factors and antibiotic resistance has been studied for years, especially in medical science. For example, in *Staphylococcus aureus*, associations between methicillin-resistance (MRSA) and virulence factors are attentively observed, as they could be responsible for very severe disease. Strains of MRSA that spread in the community have demonstrated higher virulence and an expanded set of virulence factors (with high secretion level) compared to sensitive strains [22]. Reciprocally, hospital-acquired

MRSA could be responsible for increased stimulation of immune cells leading to more severe consequences, especially when exposed to inappropriate antibiotic treatment [23]. In gram-negative bacteria, such as *Pseudomonas aeruginosa*, some studies have shown that oprD mutants (an efflux pump) were more virulent than their oprD+ counterparts in a mouse model of respiratory infections [24]. This null mutation commonly arises in clinical isolates during therapy and is associated with carbapenem resistance [25]. Infections with such isolates are associated with worse clinical outcomes, associating virulence and antibiotic resistance [26]. Finally, in *E. coli*, virulence factors located in the chromosome, such as aerobactin and fimbriae, are frequently absent in antibiotic-resistant isolates, contrarily to the ones resistant to tetracyclin (*tetA* and *tetB*-positive strains) [27–30]. On the other hand, blaCTX-M15-positive and blaOXA-2 positive UPEC isolates presented more *colV, colE2-E9, colIa-Ib, hlyA* and *csgA* genes and more *colM, colB, colE,* and *crl* genes respectively [31]. All in all, these results could highlight the difficulty to interpret results in such a highly diversified clinically-based population.

By design, non-expensive processes, e.g., agglutination assays, were applied to determine the possible interest of this determination in the routine management of the sample and of the isolated bacteria. Even if this process is not as precise as molecular biology determination processes, the description of the nature of the different genetic supports or mutations in previous studies has demonstrated the very low number of discrepant results of phenotypic agglutination compared to molecular biology. For example, the study by Kaczmarek et al. demonstrated a single discrepant result out of sixty-six tested samples, representing an exactitude of more than 98% for the agglutination assays when molecular biology is considered as a gold standard [32].

As described in Table 1, there was no over-representation of K1-positive *E. coli* prevalence compared to K1-negative strains in clinical samples. Many authors have demonstrated that the majority of neonatal meningitis cases are due to K1-positive *E. coli*, while other authors have reported that these particular strains are less frequent in vaginal tracts, in a similar proportion between pregnant and non-pregnant women [10,33–35]. Some authors have demonstrated, using DNA hybridization methods, that virulence patterns (including K1-capsules) of strains isolated from blood culture and cerebrospinal fluid were different from those of urogenital strains [36]. This observation is nowadays contested, due to similar representation, as in the present study, of K1-positive and K1 negative strains (40% and 60% approximately in the present study). Moreover, in the present study, a similar proportion of bacteremia due to *E. coli* were K1-positive or K1-negative. This observation is in contradiction with the previous observation of a difference of phenotypic characterization in blood culture for strains isolated in adults and children alike [12].

Furthermore, an insufficient number of puncture fluids was included to confirm/refute this observation, and the study is limited regarding this conclusion. Moreover, by design, and due to the clinical nature of this study and using phenotypic determination based on agglutination assays, (absence of) difference regarding the K1-antigen distribution between intestinal and extra-intestinal strains as suggested by previous publications cannot be confirmed [37].

In literal terms, "multi-drug resistant strains" (MDR) means "resistant to more than one antimicrobial agent". Nevertheless, and as stated in Magiorakos et al., this definition is not applied by Infection Control societies that consider MDR strains as gram-negative bacteria "resistant to three or more antimicrobial classes" [38]. In order to facilitate the reader's understanding, and in order to highlight the difference between the accepted notion described in this article and the present manuscript, strains resistant to at least two classes are herein considered as pluri-resistant strains. Moreover, in the present manuscript, resistance to at least one molecule within an antibiotic class was used to indicate resistance to the entire category. While this impact could be considered as a limited and crude indicator, this approach has already been used by scientific networks such as the National Healthcare Safety Network, that define, for example, carbapenem-resistance in *Klebsiella* spp. as resistance to imipenem, meropenem, ertapenem or doripenem [39,40].

Both these comments support but also temper the findings of this article, calling for greater standardization of future studies.

K1-positive strains were observed as being less frequently associated with resistance modification of at least two different antimicrobial classes. In the present study, more than half of the strains tested for AST were susceptible to all antibiotics, without any difference between groups. This proportion has previously been suggested in some studies (60% in the study by Kaczmarek et al.) and demonstrated as higher than others (14.3% for Cisowska et al.) [32,41]. Up until now, no study has had a number of strains sufficient to explore the possible association of ESBL with K1-antigen. Nevertheless, and as expected, the results have not demonstrated a possible association of this plasmid-carried mechanism of antibiotic resistance with a genomic virulence factor such as K1-antigen capsule.

The present study used only validated processes for AST phenotype determination, based on the EUCAST process and recommendations and allowing for robust comparisons to other studies. Finally, regarding specific antimicrobial classes that were associated with K1-positive or -negative strains, the study demonstrated that in this cohort, K1-negative *E. coli* presented a phenotypic profile more frequently associated with chromosomal resistance (inhibitor-resistance TEM -IRT-, mutation in *gyrA/B* or *frxA/rdxA* implicated in resistance to quinolone and Trimethoprim—sulfamethoxazole respectively) and associated with K1-negative *E. coli* strains. In pediatric samples, Fujita et al. highlighted differences between *E. coli* strains regarding susceptibility to ampicillin, with higher susceptibility in K1 positive ones, which is supported by observations by Jamie et al. using urine sampled from pregnant women with a higher susceptible proportion in K1-positive strains. Both Cisowska et al. and Nolewasjka-Lasak et al. noted a similar representation of antibiotic resistance in urinary and vaginal/cervical strains respectively [41–44].

Compared to previous publications, such as Kaczmarek et al. in 2011, which focused on bacterial strains isolated from newborns, different AST phenotypes could be observed for penicillin associated with inhibitors with higher resistance in K1-negative strains, but there was no difference on second to fourth generation cephalosporin [32]. On the contrary, the difference for Trimethoprim—sulfamethoxazole and quinolone has not been previously demonstrated, except for cotrimoxazole, by Cisowska et al., on uro-pathogenic strains only [41]. Moreover, differences could be observed for strains insensitive to at least two antimicrobial classes. This observation is supported by the study of Cole et al. in which an inverse correlation between the total number of virulence factors and non-susceptible antibiotics appears [45].

All in all, these observations highlighted that K1-determination probably cannot be used when positive as a predictable marker of pre-emptive susceptibility.

Author Contributions: Conceptualization, M.P. (Maelys Proquot), J.C. and M.P. (Maxime Pichon); methodology, C.P.-J. and M.P. (Maxime Pichon).; software, M.P. (Maxime Pichon); validation, M.P. (Maelys Proquot); L.N.J. and M.P. (Maxime Pichon); formal analysis, M.P. (Maelys Proquot); and L.N.J.; investigation, M.P. (Maelys Proquot); L.N.J.; resources, C.B. and M.P. (Maxime Pichon); data curation, M.P. (Maxime Pichon); writing—original draft preparation, M.P. (Maxime Pichon); writing—review and editing, M.P. (Maelys Proquot), L.N.J., C.P.-J., A.M., L.B., C.B., J.C. and M.P. (Maxime Pichon); visualization, M.P (Maxime Pichon); supervision, M.P. (Maxime Pichon); project administration, M.P. (Maxime Pichon); funding acquisition, M.P. (Maxime Pichon). All authors have read and agreed to the published version of the manuscript.

Funding: This research received no external funding.

Institutional Review Board Statement: The study was conducted according to the guidelines of the Declaration of Helsinki. Ethical review and approval were waived for this study, due to the retrospective nature of the study.

Informed Consent Statement: Patient consent was waived due to the retrospective nature of the study.

Data Availability Statement: Not applicable.

Acknowledgments: The authors wish to thank all laboratory technicians for their valuable help in the technical performance of these analyses and gratefully acknowledge Jeffrey Arsham, an American translator, for his rereading and revision of the original English-language manuscript.

Conflicts of Interest: The authors declare no conflict of interest regarding to the present study.

References

1. Schiffer, M.S.; Oliveira, E.; Glode, M.P.; McCracken, G.H.; Sarff, L.M.; Robbins, J.B. A Review: Relation between Invasiveness and the K1 Capsular Polysaccharide of Escherichia Coli. *Pediatr. Res.* **1976**, *10*, 82–87. [CrossRef]
2. Kauffmann, F.; Vahlne, G. About the importance of the serological change of the boron for the bacteriophage effect in the coli group. *Acta Pathol. Microbiol. Scand.* **1945**, *22*, 119–137. [CrossRef] [PubMed]
3. Bolaños, R.; DeWitt, C.W. Isolation and Characterization of the K1 (L) Antigen of Escherichia Coli. *J. Bacteriol.* **1966**, *91*, 987–996. [CrossRef]
4. Orskov, F.; Orskov, I.; Jann, B.; Jann, K. Immunoelectrophoretic Patterns of Extracts from All Escherichia Coli O and K Antigen Test Strains: Correlation with Pathogenicity. *Acta Pathol. Microbiol. Scand. B Microbiol. Immunol.* **1971**, *79*, 142–152. [CrossRef]
5. Orskov, I.; Orskov, F.; Jann, B.; Jann, K. Acidic Polysaccharide Antigens of a New Type from E.Coli Capsules. *Nature* **1963**, *200*, 144–146. [CrossRef] [PubMed]
6. Smith, D.E. Studies on Pathogenic B. Coli from Bovine Sources. IV. A Biochemical Study of the Capsular Substance. *J. Exp. Med.* **1927**, *46*, 155–166. [CrossRef]
7. Kauffmann, F. On the Significance of L Antigens for the Serology, Immunology and Pathogenicity of Escherichia Species. *Zentralbl. Bakteriol. Orig. A* **1974**, *229*, 178–189.
8. Glynn, A.A.; Brumfitt, W.; Howard, C.J. K Antigens of Escherichia Coli and Renal Involvement in Urinary-Tract Infections. *Lancet* **1971**, *1*, 514–516. [CrossRef]
9. Glynn, A.A.; Howard, C.J. The Sensitivity to Complement of Strains of Escherichia Coli Related to Their K Antigens. *Immunology* **1970**, *18*, 331–346. [PubMed]
10. Obata-Yasuoka, M.; Ba-Thein, W.; Tsukamoto, T.; Yoshikawa, H.; Hayashi, H. Vaginal Escherichia Coli Share Common Virulence Factor Profiles, Serotypes and Phylogeny with Other Extraintestinal E. coli. *Microbiology* **2002**, *148*, 2745–2752. [CrossRef]
11. Robbins, J.B.; McCracken, G.H.; Gotschlich, E.C.; Orskov, F.; Orskov, I.; Hanson, L.A. Escherichia Coli K1 Capsular Polysaccharide Associated with Neonatal Meningitis. *N. Engl. J. Med.* **1974**, *290*, 1216–1220. [CrossRef]
12. Kaijser, B. Immunology of Escherichia Coli: K Antigen and Its Relation to Urinary-Tract Infection. *J. Infect. Dis.* **1973**, *127*, 670–677. [CrossRef]
13. Kim, K.J.; Elliott, S.J.; Di Cello, F.; Stins, M.F.; Kim, K.S. The K1 Capsule Modulates Trafficking of E. Coli-Containing Vacuoles and Enhances Intracellular Bacterial Survival in Human Brain Microvascular Endothelial Cells. *Cell Microbiol.* **2003**, *5*, 245–252. [CrossRef]
14. Stins, M.F.; Prasadarao, N.V.; Ibric, L.; Wass, C.A.; Luckett, P.; Kim, K.S. Binding Characteristics of S Fimbriated Escherichia Coli to Isolated Brain Microvascular Endothelial Cells. *Am. J. Pathol.* **1994**, *145*, 1228–1236. [PubMed]
15. Mekalanos, J.J. Environmental Signals Controlling Expression of Virulence Determinants in Bacteria. *J. Bacteriol.* **1992**, *174*, 1–7. [CrossRef] [PubMed]
16. Bingen-Bidois, M.; Clermont, O.; Bonacorsi, S.; Terki, M.; Brahimi, N.; Loukil, C.; Barraud, D.; Bingen, E. Phylogenetic Analysis and Prevalence of Urosepsis Strains of Escherichia Coli Bearing Pathogenicity Island-like Domains. *Infect. Immun.* **2002**, *70*, 3216–3226. [CrossRef] [PubMed]
17. Jain, A.; Roy, I.; Gupta, M.K.; Kumar, M.; Agarwal, S.K. Prevalence of Extended-Spectrum Beta-Lactamase-Producing Gram-Negative Bacteria in Septicaemic Neonates in a Tertiary Care Hospital. *J. Med. Microbiol.* **2003**, *52*, 421–425. [CrossRef]
18. Schrag, S.J.; Farley, M.M.; Petit, S.; Reingold, A.; Weston, E.J.; Pondo, T.; Hudson Jain, J.; Lynfield, R. Epidemiology of Invasive Early-Onset Neonatal Sepsis, 2005 to 2014. *Pediatrics* **2016**, *138*, e20162013. [CrossRef]
19. Huynh, B.-T.; Padget, M.; Garin, B.; Herindrainy, P.; Kermorvant-Duchemin, E.; Watier, L.; Guillemot, D.; Delarocque-Astagneau, E. Burden of Bacterial Resistance among Neonatal Infections in Low Income Countries: How Convincing Is the Epidemiological Evidence? *BMC Infect. Dis.* **2015**, *15*, 127. [CrossRef] [PubMed]
20. Mendoza-Palomar, N.; Balasch-Carulla, M.; González-Di Lauro, S.; Céspedes, M.C.; Andreu, A.; Frick, M.A.; Linde, M.A.; Soler-Palacin, P. Escherichia Coli Early-Onset Sepsis: Trends over Two Decades. *Eur. J. Pediatr.* **2017**, *176*, 1227–1234. [CrossRef]
21. Weissman, S.J.; Hansen, N.I.; Zaterka-Baxter, K.; Higgins, R.D.; Stoll, B.J. Emergence of Antibiotic Resistance-Associated Clones Among Escherichia Coli Recovered From Newborns With Early-Onset Sepsis and Meningitis in the United States, 2008–2009. *J. Pediatric Infect. Dis. Soc.* **2016**, *5*, 269–276. [CrossRef]
22. Cameron, D.R.; Howden, B.P.; Peleg, A.Y. The Interface between Antibiotic Resistance and Virulence in Staphylococcus Aureus and Its Impact upon Clinical Outcomes. *Clin. Infect. Dis.* **2011**, *53*, 576–582. [CrossRef] [PubMed]
23. Gasch, O.; Camoez, M.; Domínguez, M.A.; Padilla, B.; Pintado, V.; Almirante, B.; Lepe, J.A.; Lagarde, M.; Ruiz de Gopegui, E.; Martínez, J.A.; et al. Predictive Factors for Early Mortality among Patients with Methicillin-Resistant Staphylococcus Aureus Bacteraemia. *J. Antimicrob. Chemother.* **2013**, *68*, 1423–1430. [CrossRef]
24. Roux, D.; Danilchanka, O.; Guillard, T.; Cattoir, V.; Aschard, H.; Fu, Y.; Angoulvant, F.; Messika, J.; Ricard, J.-D.; Mekalanos, J.J.; et al. Fitness Cost of Antibiotic Susceptibility during Bacterial Infection. *Sci. Transl. Med.* **2015**, *7*, 297ra114. [CrossRef] [PubMed]

25. Skurnik, D.; Roux, D.; Cattoir, V.; Danilchanka, O.; Lu, X.; Yoder-Himes, D.R.; Han, K.; Guillard, T.; Jiang, D.; Gaultier, C.; et al. Enhanced in Vivo Fitness of Carbapenem-Resistant OprD Mutants of Pseudomonas Aeruginosa Revealed through High-Throughput Sequencing. *Proc. Natl. Acad. Sci. USA* **2013**, *110*, 20747–20752. [CrossRef] [PubMed]
26. Peña, C.; Suarez, C.; Gozalo, M.; Murillas, J.; Almirante, B.; Pomar, V.; Aguilar, M.; Granados, A.; Calbo, E.; Rodríguez-Baño, J.; et al. Prospective Multicenter Study of the Impact of Carbapenem Resistance on Mortality in Pseudomonas Aeruginosa Bloodstream Infections. *Antimicrob. Agents Chemother.* **2012**, *56*, 1265–1272. [CrossRef]
27. Karami, N.; Nowrouzian, F.; Adlerberth, I.; Wold, A.E. Tetracycline Resistance in Escherichia Coli and Persistence in the Infantile Colonic Microbiota. *Antimicrob. Agents Chemother.* **2006**, *50*, 156–161. [CrossRef] [PubMed]
28. Johnson, J.R.; Moseley, S.L.; Roberts, P.L.; Stamm, W.E. Aerobactin and Other Virulence Factor Genes among Strains of Escherichia Coli Causing Urosepsis: Association with Patient Characteristics. *Infect. Immun.* **1988**, *56*, 405–412. [CrossRef]
29. Horcajada, J.P.; Soto, S.; Gajewski, A.; Smithson, A.; Jiménez de Anta, M.T.; Mensa, J.; Vila, J.; Johnson, J.R. Quinolone-Resistant Uropathogenic Escherichia Coli Strains from Phylogenetic Group B2 Have Fewer Virulence Factors than Their Susceptible Counterparts. *J. Clin. Microbiol.* **2005**, *43*, 2962–2964. [CrossRef]
30. Liu, X.; Liu, H.; Li, Y.; Hao, C. Association between Virulence Profile and Fluoroquinolone Resistance in Escherichia Coli Isolated from Dogs and Cats in China. *J. Infect. Dev. Ctries* **2017**, *11*, 306–313. [CrossRef]
31. Abd El-Baky, R.M.; Ibrahim, R.A.; Mohamed, D.S.; Ahmed, E.F.; Hashem, Z.S. Prevalence of Virulence Genes and Their Association with Antimicrobial Resistance Among Pathogenic E. Coli Isolated from Egyptian Patients with Different Clinical Infections. *Infect. Drug Resist.* **2020**, *13*, 1221–1236. [CrossRef]
32. Kaczmarek, A.; Budzyńska, A.; Gospodarek, E. Detection of K1 Antigen of Escherichia Coli Rods Isolated from Pregnant Women and Neonates. *Folia Microbiol.* **2014**, *59*, 419–422. [CrossRef]
33. Kim, K.S. Pathogenesis of Bacterial Meningitis: From Bacteraemia to Neuronal Injury. *Nat. Rev. Neurosci.* **2003**, *4*, 376–385. [CrossRef] [PubMed]
34. Watt, S.; Lanotte, P.; Mereghetti, L.; Moulin-Schouleur, M.; Picard, B.; Quentin, R. Escherichia Coli Strains from Pregnant Women and Neonates: Intraspecies Genetic Distribution and Prevalence of Virulence Factors. *J. Clin. Microbiol.* **2003**, *41*, 1929–1935. [CrossRef]
35. Korhonen, T.K.; Valtonen, M.V.; Parkkinen, J.; Väisänen-Rhen, V.; Finne, J.; Orskov, F.; Orskov, I.; Svenson, S.B.; Mäkelä, P.H. Serotypes, Hemolysin Production, and Receptor Recognition of Escherichia Coli Strains Associated with Neonatal Sepsis and Meningitis. *Infect. Immun.* **1985**, *48*, 486–491. [CrossRef]
36. Bollmann, R.; Seeburg, A.; Parschau, J.; Schönian, G.; Sokolowska-Köhler, W.; Halle, E.; Presber, W. Genotypic and Phenotypic Determination of Five Virulence Markers in Clinical Isolates of Escherichia Coli. *FEMS Immunol. Med. Microbiol.* **1997**, *17*, 263–271. [CrossRef]
37. Ananias, M.; Yano, T. Serogroups and Virulence Genotypes of Escherichia Coli Isolated from Patients with Sepsis. *Braz. J. Med. Biol. Res.* **2008**, *41*, 877–883. [CrossRef] [PubMed]
38. Magiorakos, A.-P.; Srinivasan, A.; Carey, R.B.; Carmeli, Y.; Falagas, M.E.; Giske, C.G.; Harbarth, S.; Hindler, J.F.; Kahlmeter, G.; Olsson-Liljequist, B.; et al. Multidrug-Resistant, Extensively Drug-Resistant and Pandrug-Resistant Bacteria: An International Expert Proposal for Interim Standard Definitions for Acquired Resistance. *Clin. Microbiol. Infect.* **2012**, *18*, 268–281. [CrossRef] [PubMed]
39. Hidron, A.I.; Edwards, J.R.; Patel, J.; Horan, T.C.; Sievert, D.M.; Pollock, D.A.; Fridkin, S.K.; National Healthcare Safety Network Team. Participating National Healthcare Safety Network Facilities NHSN Annual Update: Antimicrobial-Resistant Pathogens Associated with Healthcare-Associated Infections: Annual Summary of Data Reported to the National Healthcare Safety Network at the Centers for Disease Control and Prevention, 2006–2007. *Infect. Control Hosp. Epidemiol.* **2008**, *29*, 996–1011. [CrossRef] [PubMed]
40. Kallen, A.J.; Hidron, A.I.; Patel, J.; Srinivasan, A. Multidrug Resistance among Gram-Negative Pathogens That Caused Healthcare-Associated Infections Reported to the National Healthcare Safety Network, 2006-2008. *Infect. Control Hosp. Epidemiol.* **2010**, *31*, 528–531. [CrossRef] [PubMed]
41. Cisowska, A.; Lewczyk, E.; Korzekwa, K.; Wojnicz, D.; Jankowski, S.; Doroszkiewicz, W. Evaluation of sensitivity to antibiotics of microorganisms isolated from children with urinary tract infections. *Pol. Merkur. Lekarski* **2003**, *14*, 322–326.
42. Fujita, K.; Yoshioka, H.; Sakata, H.; Murono, K.; Kakehashi, H.; Kaeriyama, M.; Tsukamoto, T. K1 Antigen, Serotype and Antibiotic Susceptibility of Escherichia Coli Isolated from Cerebrospinal Fluid, Blood and Other Specimens from Japanese Infants. *Acta Paediatr. Jpn.* **1990**, *32*, 610–614. [CrossRef] [PubMed]
43. Nolewajka-Lasak, I.; Rajca, M.; Kamiński, K.; Kunicka, M.; Król, W. Antibiotic sensitivity of Enterobacteriaceae isolated from women vagina and uterine cervix. *Med. Dosw. Mikrobiol.* **2003**, *55*, 351–356. [PubMed]
44. Jamie, W.E.; Edwards, R.K.; Duff, P. Antimicrobial Susceptibility of Gram-Negative Uropathogens Isolated from Obstetric Patients. *Infect. Dis. Obstet. Gynecol.* **2002**, *10*, 123–126. [CrossRef] [PubMed]
45. Cole, B.K.; Ilikj, M.; McCloskey, C.B.; Chavez-Bueno, S. Antibiotic Resistance and Molecular Characterization of Bacteremia Escherichia Coli Isolates from Newborns in the United States. *PLoS ONE* **2019**, *14*, e0219352. [CrossRef]

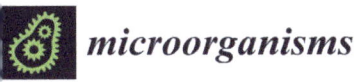

Article

Escherichia coli Specific Virulence-Gene Markers Analysis for Quality Control of Ovine Cheese in Slovakia

Dobroslava Bujňáková *, Lívia Karahutová and Vladimír Kmeť

Centre of Biosciences of the Slovak Academy of Sciences, Institute of Animal Physiology, 04001 Košice, Slovakia; karahutova@saske.sk (L.K.); kmetv@saske.sk (V.K.)
* Correspondence: dbujnak@saske.sk

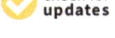

Abstract: Shiga toxin-producing and extra-intestinal pathogenic *Escherichia coli* (*E. coli*) have the potential to spread through faecal waste, resulting in contamination of food and causing foodborne disease outbreaks. With the aim of characterizing unpasteurized ovine cheese in Slovakia, a total of 92 *E. coli* strains were examined for eleven representative virulence genes typical for (extra-)intestinal pathogenic *E. coli* and phylogenetic grouping. Phylogenetic groups B1 (36%) and A (32%) were the most dominant, followed by groups C (14%) and D (13%), while the lowest incidence was recorded for F (4%), and E (1%), and 43 (47%) samples carried at least one virulent gene, i.e., potential pathogens. Isolates present in groups E, F and D showed higher presence of virulence genes (100%, 75%, and 67%), versus 55%, 39%, and 28% in commensal B1, C, and A, respectively. Occurrence of *papC* and *fyuA* (both 24%) was highest, followed by *tsh*, *iss*, *stx2*, *cnf1*, *kpsII*, *cvaC*, *stx1*, *iutA* and *eaeA*. Nine *E. coli* strains (almost 10% of all tested and around 21% of our virulence-gene-associated isolates) harboured *stx1*, *stx2* or *eae*. Ovine cheeses in Slovakia are highly contaminated with *E. coli* including potentially pathogenic strains capable of causing intestinal and/or extra-intestinal diseases, and thus may pose a threat to public health while unpasteurized.

Keywords: ExPEC; STEC; pathogenic potential; phylogenetic grouping; PCR

Citation: Bujňáková, D.; Karahutová, L.; Kmeť, V. *Escherichia coli* Specific Virulence-Gene Markers Analysis for Quality Control of Ovine Cheese in Slovakia. *Microorganisms* **2021**, *9*, 1808. https://doi.org/10.3390/microorganisms9091808

Academic Editor: Sangryeol Ryu

Received: 23 July 2021
Accepted: 24 August 2021
Published: 25 August 2021

Publisher's Note: MDPI stays neutral with regard to jurisdictional claims in published maps and institutional affiliations.

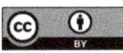

Copyright: © 2021 by the authors. Licensee MDPI, Basel, Switzerland. This article is an open access article distributed under the terms and conditions of the Creative Commons Attribution (CC BY) license (https://creativecommons.org/licenses/by/4.0/).

1. Introduction

Public health hazards associated with consumption of unpasteurized milk products, including related foodborne disease outbreaks, have been reported in parts of the world [1,2], and consequently strict control of the microbial quality of these types of food is required.

Dairy products can be contaminated with various bacteria. Among the pathogenic agents, *Listeria monocytogenes*, *Salmonella* spp., Shiga toxin-producing *E. coli* (STEC) serotype O157:H7 and enterotoxin-producing *Staphylococcus aureus* are most involved in foodborne outbreaks related to the consumption of raw milk cheese in industrialized countries [3]. These foodborne pathogens usually cause illness with acute symptoms restricted to the gastrointestinal tract. However, in some cases, they can cause serious extra-intestinal diseases such as Hemolytic Uremic Syndrome (HUS) associated with *E. coli* O157:H7 [4].

The authors Cancino-Padilla et al. [5] compiled a summary of outbreaks associated with the consumption of various dairy products in the world. Several outbreaks have been associated with the consumption of cheese and other ready to-eat foods concerning their main contaminant *E. coli* stemming from faecal or farm environmental contamination during the milking process [6,7].

The presence of *E. coli* as a reliable indicator of direct or indirect poisoning testifies not only to poor hygienic practices but also (and worse) it can be a source of virulence genes rendering the bacteria pathogenic with the ability to cause a variety of sicknesses. *E. coli* associated with animal or human diseases are divided into two major groups, intestinal and extra-intestinal, and based on their virulence properties into several subgroups (intestinal: enteropathogenic *E. coli* (EPEC), enterohemorrhagic *E. coli* (EHEC) or Shiga toxin-producing *E. coli* (STEC), enterotoxigenic *E. coli* (ETEC), enteroinvasive *E. coli* (EIEC), enteroaggregative *E. coli* (EAEC), and diffusely adherent *E. coli* (DAEC); extra-intestinal: uropathogenic *E. coli* (UPEC), avian pathogenic *E. coli* (APEC), meningitis-associated *E. coli* (MNEC) and necrotoxigenic *E. coli* (NTEC)) [8]. Moreover, virulence-hybrid *E. coli* isolates have also been reported [9,10].

Virulence factors (VF) related to the pathogenicity of various subtypes of *E. coli* are numerous and have a wide range of activity, from those enabled for bacteria colonization to those causing virulence, including adhesins, toxins, iron acquisition factors and polysaccharide capsules, which are usually encoded on pathogenicity islands (PAIs), plasmids and other mobile genetic elements. The most important PAI in Enterobacterales is High Pathogenicity Island, encoded primarily in the iron-uptake system essential for enhancing bacterial condition, the so-called "fitness cost". Iron uptake as an important survival factor, along with resistance and virulence, allows bacteria to establish in a competitive environment [11].

Since healthy adult cattle and sheep are an asymptomatic reservoir of STEC, faecal contaminating *E. coli* strains isolated from milk and dairy products often contain high prevalence of Vero or Shiga-toxins (*vtx1* and *vtx2* or *stx1* and *stx2*), intimin (*eaeA*) and hemolysin (*hlyA*). These factors can cause bacterial adhesion and invasion into the intestinal epithelial cells, causing severe attaching-effacing (A/E) lesions. Certain STEC occurrence in raw milk, in the particular serotype O157:H7, is well documented and represents a concern since up to 10% of people infected with these bacteria develop HUS, which is potentially a lethal condition, especially in children, immune-deficient and elderly people [12,13]. In 2018, EFSA (European Food Safety Authority) reported a total of 5079 foodborne outbreaks of which 14, involving 775 people, were linked to cheese consumption, and the most common causative agents were STEC and bacterial toxins [14]. The results obtained so far point to the importance of food vehicles in the diffusion of STEC infections at the EU level. Analysis of the virulence gene profiles of the isolated STEC strains highlights the presence of STEC in food with potential for causing severe disease. EFSA recommends reporting on the STEC virulence genes as their analysis represents the basis for molecular risk assessment and the most valuable tool for predicting that risk and the severity of STEC infections in humans.

In recent years, investigators have hypothesized that food, including unpasteurized milk products, can be a reservoir for many other virulence factors responsible for extra-intestinal infections, and can play a major role in the transmission of ExPEC (Extraintestinal pathogenic *Escherichia coli*) strains [2,15,16]. Although research has been ongoing for many years, specific criteria for classifying *E. coli* strains such as ExPEC have not so far been established. According to results obtained by Johnson and Russo [17], ExPEC were defined as *E. coli* isolates containing two or more virulence markers, which were identified by means of multiplex PCR reaction, including *papA* genes (a structural subunit of P-fimbriae) and/or *papC* (P fimbriae), *sfa/foc* (S and F1C fimbriae subunits), *afa/dra* (adhesins binding antigen Dr), *kpsMT II* (group 2 capsular polysaccharides) and *iutA* (aerobactin receptor) [18]. However, for many bacterial pathogens infecting mucosal tissues, expression of only one specific adhesin is critical and sufficient for pathogenesis. Disruption of the ability of a bacterial pathogen to attach and to colonize a specific tissue by adhesin-mediated receptor recognition is often enough to make it avirulent [2].

Bearing in mind that the possibility of transmission of various pathogenic intestinal and extra-intestinal *E. coli* strains to humans, causing diseases through consumption of raw milk as well as raw milk products, has been reported worldwide [19,20], monitoring not only of *E. coli* presence, but also their pathogenic potential through virulence genes occurrence, becomes a significant necessity. With regard to this development and due to the paucity of data on the microbial contamination of cheese, mainly concerning virulence-associated genes and phylogenetic distribution in Slovakia, we examined 92 *E. coli* isolates from unpasteurized ovine cheeses for possession of traits associated with the virulence of human extra-intestinal pathogenic *E. coli* (ExPEC) or intestinal Vero (Shiga) toxin (*Vtx* or

Stx)-producing *E. coli* (VTEC or STEC): e.g., *iutA*, *iss*, *cvaC*, *kpsII*, *tsh*, *papC*, *fyuA*, *cnf1*, *stx1*, *stx2*, *eaeA* and phylogenetic grouping.

2. Materials and Methods

2.1. Source of Samples and Isolation

During the course of one year (August 2018–August 2019), 92 samples of ovine cheese were obtained from local farmers in western Slovakia. The samples were collected in sterile sample collection bags transferred to the laboratory in a cool-box. All cheese samples showed normal physical character including consistency, odour and colour. Ten grams of each cheese sample were homogenized in a Stomacher (BioTech, Prague, Czech Republic) with 90 mL of sterile buffered peptone water (Oxoid, Basingstoke, UK). After preparing the 1:10 dilution, samples were streaked onto Mac Conkey Agar (Oxoid, Basingstoke, UK) and UriSelect Agar (Bio-Rad Laboratories, Hercules, CA, USA) overnight at 37 °C. The typical colonies on both agars were isolated, identified and confirmed as *E. coli* using MALDI-TOF MS biotyper (Bruker Daltonics, Bremen, Germany) [21] and ENTEROtest24 (Erba Lachema Brno, Czech Republic). A single colony of *E. coli* was isolated from each sample.

2.2. DNA Preparation

The cultures were inoculated on Nutrient Agar (Oxoid, Basingstoke, UK) and incubated at 37 °C for 24 h. A bacteriological loop was used to carry part of the colony into 100 µL distilled water, which was then vortexed, boiled for 10 min and centrifuged for 2 min at $12,000 \times g$, and the supernatant was used for PCR.

2.3. Phylogenetic Groups

All isolates were assigned to phylogenetic groups (A, B1, C, B2, D, E and F) based on Clermont phylogenetic typing schemes [22]. The protocols are based on amplification of *chuA*, *yjaA*, *arpA*, *TspE4.C2* DNA fragments and additional testing for specific genes in the E (*arpAgpE*) and C (*trpAgpC*) groups. Classification of the strains was performed based on the presence or absence of genes.

2.4. Genes of Virulence Factors

All isolates were subjected to a multiplex and/or single PCR analysis for detection genes associated with ExPEC, specifically: *iutA*–receptor for aerobactin, *cvaC*–colicin V, *kpsII*–capsular polysialic acid virulence factor, *iss*–increased serum survival, *tsh*–temperature sensitive haemagglutinin, *papC*–P fimbrial adhesin and *fyuA*–yersiniabactin receptor for ferric yersiniabactin uptake. Moreover, we used genes encoding Shiga-toxin types 1, 2 (*stx1*, *stx2*), cytotoxic necrotizing factor (CNF1) and the gene encoding intimin for attaching and effacing mechanisms (*eaeA*). PCR primers, length of their amplified products, annealing and references are listed in Table 1. The amplifications were carried out in a single tube with a volume of 25 µL, utilizing TaqI polymerase (Solis Biodyne, Tartu, Estonia). Amplified products were run on 1.5% agarose gel.

Table 1. PCR primers, length of the amplified products, annealing and references.

Gene	Primer Sequence (5'3')	Product	T_{ann}	Reference
arpA	AACGCTATTCGCCAGCTTGC TCTCCCCATACCGTACGCTA	400 bp	59 °C	[22]
chuA	ATGGTACCGGACGAACCAAC TGCCGCCAGTACCAAAGACA	288 bp	59 °C	[22]
yjaA	CAAACGTGAAGTGTCAGGAG AATGCGTTCCTCAACCTGTG	211 bp	59 °C	[22]
tspE4.C4	CACTATTCGTAAGGTCATCC AGTTTATCGCTGCGGGTCGC	152 bp	59 °C	[22]

Table 1. Cont.

Gene	Primer Sequence (5'3')	Product	T_{ann}	Reference
ArpAgpE.f	GATTCCATCTTGTCAAAATATGCC GAAAAGAAAAAGAATTCCCAAGAG	301 bp	57 °C	[23]
trpAgpC.1	AGTTTTATGCCCAGTGCGAG TCTGCGCCGGTCACGCCC	219 bp	59 °C	[23]
kps II	GCGCATTTGCTGATACTGTTG CATCCAGACGATAAGCATGAGCA	272 bp	63 °C	[24]
iss	ATCACATAGGATTCTGCCG ACAAAAAGTTCTATCGCTTCC	700 bp	61 °C	[25]
papC	GACGGCTGTACTGCAGGGTGTGGCG ATATCCTTTCTGCAGGGATGCAATA	328 bp	61 °C	[26]
cvaC	CACACACAAACGGGAGCTGTT CACACACAAACGGGAGCTGTT	680 bp	63 °C	[24]
tsh	GGTGGTGCACTGGAGTGG AGTCCAGCGTGATAGTGG	620 bp	55 °C	[27]
iutA	GGCTGGACATGGGAACTGG CGTCGGGAACGGGTAGAATCG	300 bp	63 °C	[24]
fyuA	TGATTAACCCCGCGACGGGAA CGCAGTAGGCACGATGTTGTA	880 bp	55 °C	[24]
stx1	ACGTTACAGCGTGTTGCRGGGATC TTGCCACAGACTGCGTCAGTRAGG	121 bp	63 °C	[28]
stx2	TGTGGCTGGGTTCGTTAATACGGC TCCGTTGTCATGGAAACCGTTGTC	102 bp	63 °C	[28]
eaeA	TGAGCGGCTGGCATGAGTCATAC TCGATCCCCATCGTCACCAGAGG	241 bp	63 °C	[28]
cnf1	GGCGACAAATGCAGTATTGCTTGG GACGTTGGTTGCGGTAATTTTGGG	552 bp	63 °C	[28]

3. Results

3.1. Phylogenetic Grouping

Phylogenetic grouping of 92 E. coli isolates from unpasteurized cheese showed that 33 (35.87%), 29 (31.52%), and 13 (14.13%) belonged in phylogenetic groups B1, A, and C respectively, as shown in Table 2, and these were followed by group D (12 isolates; 13.04%). Finally, groups E and F were less prevalent with 1.09% (1 isolate) and 4.35% (4 isolates), while group B2 was not detected.

Table 2. Phylogenetic distribution of E. coli from unpasteurized cheese.

Phylogenetic Groups	No. of Isolates/% of Occurrence (n = 92)	Distribution According to Gene Groupings (n)	Quadruplex Genotype and Next Step for C or E Phylogroup					
			arpA	chuA	yjaA	TspE4.C4	ArpA for E Group	trpA for C Group
Group A/C	29/(32%)	12	+					
		17	+		+			-
Group C	13/(14%)	13	+		+			+
Group B1	33/(36%)	33	+			+		
Group D/E	12/(13%)	8	+	+		+	-	
		4	+	+			-	
Group E	1/(1%)	1	+	+	+		+	
Group F	4/(4%)	4		+				

Phylogenetic groups B1 and A were predominant among the tested isolates. It is interesting to note that 54.6% (18/33) of isolates belonging in group B1 as well as 100% (1/1), 75% (3/4) and 66.6% (8/12) of isolates belonging in groups E, F and D respectively, were found to have at least one of the examined virulence genes (four isolates contained three virulence genes—*iss, cvaC, papC*— group B1; *iss, iutA, cnf1*— group D; *stx1, stx2, cnf1*—group B1 and *iss, cvaC, cnf1*-group C) (Tables 3 and 4).

Table 3. The percentage of occurrence of virulence-related genes in various phylogenetic groups of *E. coli*.

Phylogenetic Groups	No. of Isolates/No. with Virulence Genes (% Virulent Strains)	Presence of Virulence Genes										
		iss	*cvaC*	*papC*	*iutA*	*tsh*	*fyuA*	*kpsII*	*stx1*	*stx2*	*eaeA*	*cnf1*
Group A	29/8 (27.6%)			1		1	4	2		2		
Group B1	33/18 (54.6%)	4	3	5	1	6	3		2	3		2
Group C	13/5 (38.5%)	1	1	2		1	1			1		2
Group D	12/8 (66.6%)	1		2	1	2	1	2	1			2
Group E	1/1 (100%)										1	
Group F	4/3 (75%)	1		1			2	1				
TOTAL	92/43 (46.7%)	7	4	11	2	10	11	5	3	6	1	6

Table 4. Presence of virulence gene patterns in *E. coli*.

No. of Genes	Virulence Genes	No. of Isolates (*n* = 92)
1	*iss*	1
1	*cvaC*	1
1	*papC*	5
1	*iutA*	1
1	*tsh*	6
1	*fyuA*	6
2	*fyuA, cnf1*	1
1	*cnf1*	1
1	*kpsII*	2
3	*iss, cvaC, cnf1*	1
2	*iss, papC*	1
2	*iss, cnf1*	1
3	*iss, iutA, cnf1*	1
2	*iss, fyuA*	1
3	*iss, cvaC, papC*	1
2	*tsh, fyuA*	1
2	*tsh, kpsII*	1
2	*tsh, stx2*	2
2	*papC, cvaC*	1
2	*papC, kpsII*	1
2	*papC, stx1*	1
2	*papC, stx2*	1
2	*fyuA, kpsII*	1
2	*fyuA, stx2*	1

Table 4. Cont.

No. of Genes	Virulence Genes	No. of Isolates (n = 92)
1	eaeA	1
1	stx1	1
1	stx2	1
3	stx1, stx2, cnf1	1
0	No gene	49

3.2. The Occurrence of E. coli and Virulence Genes in Unpasteurized Cheese

All 92 samples of ovine cheese collected from various locations in western Slovakia were contaminated with *E. coli*. Isolates were investigated for the presence of 11 virulence genes usually present in pathogenic *E. coli*. The occurrence of potentially pathogenic *E. coli* (which carried one or more of the targeted virulence genes) was 47% (n = 43). The remaining 49 (53%) isolates were negative. Isolates present in groups E, F and D showed the highest presence of virulence genes (100%, 75% and 67% respectively); however phylogenetic groups considered as commensal, i.e., B1, C and A, also had a high incidence of virulence genes (55%, 39% and 28% respectively). It was found that the most prevalent genes among 43 isolates with virulence factors were *papC* and *fyuA* detected in 11 isolates (both 51%), while 10 (23%), 7 (16%), 6 (14%), 6 (14%), 5 (12%), 4 (9%), 3 (7%), 2 (4.6%) and 1 (2.3%) isolates were positive for *tsh, iss, stx2, cnf1, kpsII, cvaC, stx1, iutA* and *eaeA* genes, respectively (Table 3).

Based on the distribution of the various virulence genes investigated, all the tested isolates exhibited 28 different virulence gene patterns. Four isolates were positive for three targeted virulence genes, 14 showed presence of two genes, and in 26 others one gene was detected.

The three most prevalent patterns consisted of isolates possessing one virulence gene, *fyuA, tsh*, or *papC* (n = 6, n = 6, n = 6 and n = 5 respectively). Based on the distribution of verotoxines and intimin, nine of the tested isolates exhibited a positive signal for one of those genes. Specifically, five isolates harbored clinically and epidemiologically the most important *stx2* alone, two only *stx1*, and one strain featured both *stx1* and *stx2* genes together with gene cnf1. The gene encoding cytotoxic necrotizing factor (CNF1) was detected in six isolates. Only one of the isolates was positive for *eae*, which could be classified as EPEC defined as *Stx*-negative *E. coli* able to produce A/E lesions on intestinal cells. Detailed results are shown in Table 4.

4. Discussion

Foodborne diseases caused by various bacterial pathogens are a significant global public health concern. Based on the above, the EU has recently strengthened the rules for strict control of food safety and public health to cope with the spread of certain infectious diseases.

The presence of *E. coli* in milk and milk products is an important indicator of faecal or environmental contamination and poor hygienic practices. Conventional microbiological diagnostics in food control include only determination of *E. coli* numbers per gram without any other characterization of isolated strains.

In addition to the presence of *E. coli* denoting faecal contamination, the presence of virulence-related genes in *E. coli* strains refers to the pathogenicity of the isolates. Previous studies documented the equation of some *E. coli* isolates from raw milk and products for virulence markers [2,19,29]. Considering the above, the present study thus aimed to assess raw cheese quality by capturing live *E. coli* and investigating the *E. coli* isolates for certain functioning virulence-associated genes using PCR assay.

Based on our results it is clear that single or double virulence factors were demonstrated in the majority of examined isolates. One isolate carried two virulence factors *papC* and *kpsII*, which were described by Johnson and Russo [17] as ExPEC, but the importance of this remains irrelevant regarding the possibility of the presence of other markers, which were not the subject of this study.

In our project, every sample of the 92 cheeses was contaminated with *E. coli*. A similar high prevalence of *E. coli* in cheese has also been reported in Brazil (96–97.7%) [20]. Altogether, 47% (43/92) of the investigated dairy products carried potentially pathogenic *E. coli* (possessing one or more of the virulence genes tested), as shown in Table 3.

When interpreting the results, keep in mind that the data of the various diagnostic procedures are not directly comparable due to differences in strategy sampling and analytical application method. Our approach used for selecting the colonies forming the dataset was based on the selection of only a single colony from every sample. A different approach was used by Skočková et al. [30] for monitoring of the occurrence of STEC in swabs from the carcasses of pigs and cattle at slaughterhouses in the Czech Republic. After homogenization and incubation, 1 mL of bacterial suspension was used for DNA isolation, and after PCR, *stx*-positive samples were inoculated on selective media, incubated overnight and up to 50 colonies from one sample with *E. coli* morphology were investigated for the presence of *stx* and *eaeA* genes. Their results showed the prevalence of STEC in cattle (3.9%) and pig (5.1%) carcasses in the Czech Republic, although raw meat has not been considered an important source of STEC.

From our results concerning *stx* and *eae*, nine *E. coli* strains (almost 10% of all tested and around 21% of our virulence gene-associated isolates) harboured *stx1*, *stx2* or *eae* (Table 4). Of these, five contained *stx2* alone, and as described by Friedrich et al. [31], *stx2* is clinically and epidemiologically the most important Shiga-toxin type, and the probability of HUS development in infections from strains harbouring *stx2* is higher than that from strains containing either *stx1* or both *stx1* and *stx2*. Healthy sheep are asymptomatic reservoirs of STEC and thus faecal contamination during milk processing explains the occurrence of these bacteria in dairy products, and this is a significant problem not only for fresh cheese, but also for hard ripened cheeses, because of the ability of STEC to survive during the production procedure with periods of maturation.

In the period 2012–2017, a total of 330 STEC outbreaks were reported in 18 countries of the European Union, involving 2841 cases, 463 hospitalizations and five fatalities. Of all these outbreaks reported, the food vehicle was identified for 164 outbreaks (49.7%) and five outbreaks by strength of evidence of identification of food vehicle were reported from Slovakia and Poland [32]. In 2018, STEC diseases were the fourth most common zoonosis in Europe.

The report on zoonosis in Slovakia indicates, that in 2016, from 46 examined food samples (cheeses from unpasteurized milk, meat products), STECs were confirmed in 28.26%. A year later, twenty-six foods were examined with only one being STEC-positive. Reports from the following years (2018–2020) did not contain data on the STEC situation in Slovakia (https://www.mpsr.sk/?navID=47&sID=111&navID2=506, accessed on 12 December 2016).

Other important virulence determinants include the locus of enterocyte effacement (LEE) shared by EPEC. This 35–45 kb pathogenicity island is responsible for the formation of attaching and effacing (A/E) lesions on intestinal epithelial cells. It contains the *eaeA* gene encoding the outer membrane adhesin, intimin, which mediates tight contact between STEC or EPEC and intestinal epithelial cells. The *eaeA* gene is a well-known virulence factor not only for EPEC and EHEC but also atypical EPEC, in which the *eaeA* gene occurs alone without the presence of adherence factor plasmid (*pEAF*) genes [8]. Our study identified the *eaeA* gene in one isolate (2.3%) (Tables 3 and 4), which could be classified as EPEC, defined as a *Stx*-negative *E. coli* strain able to produce A/E lesions on intestinal cells, detectable in vitro by means of positive *eae* PCR testing. Our result showing the occurrence of the *eae* gene is in agreement with several previous studies: 9.1% in Saudi Arabia [19], 3.1% in Slovakia [29] and 0.9% in Egypt [2].

Since none of our strains carried *stx* and *eae* together, the strains would not have to be able to adhere to the cells and produce Shiga toxins. However, the EFSA Journal [32] notes, inter alia, that the presence of intimin (*eae* gene) was an aggravating factor, but this virulence factor was not always essential for severe illness, suggesting that there is an alternative mechanism of attachment. As an example, during 2011, a large outbreak caused by an unusual *E. coli* strain was reported in Germany. The pathotype combined the virulence potential of STEC and enteroaggregative *E. coli*. The aggregative adherence fimbriae colonization mechanism substituted for the locus of enterocyte effacement functions normally encoded by the *eae* gene in EHEC strains. Clinical presentation of the infection also included bloody diarrhea and HUS [33]. The Cytotoxic Necrotizing Factor (CNF1) [28] is a bacterial virulence factor associated with ExPEC strains causing urinary tract infection and meningitis that induces a drastic rebuilding of the microfilamental network on various eukaryotic cells in culture into thick stress fibers. The *cnf1* was detected in six (6.5%) of all tested and around 14% of our virulence-gene-associated isolates. The incidence of the *cnf1* virulence marker in *E. coli* strains isolated from traditional Slovak ovine cheese was also described by Holko et al. [29], and *cnf1* was confirmed in 3 isolates from 95 (3%) examined overall.

Other occurring virulence-associated traits were genes for adhesins, protectins/serum resistance, iron uptake and toxins: *papC*, *iss*, *cvaC*, *kpsII*, *fyuA*, *iutA* and *tsh*-specific virulence markers associated with extra-intestinal infection. One of the explanations for their occurrence in milk and dairy products could be the possibility of udder infection (pre/sub-clinical mastitis) [34].

Of the adhesion- and iron uptake-encoding virulence factors included in our study, the *papC* and *fyuA* genes were the most frequent. We found 11 *E. coli* harbouring *papC* (P fimbria), a gene which has been associated with upper urinary tract infection [35], and in some isolates was associated with some of the genes under investigation in this study: *iss*, *cvaC*, *kpsII*, *stx1* and/or *stx2*. A combination of P fimbria and Shiga-toxins could be interesting due to the possibility of their causing problems related to urinary tract infection and HUS. Eleven of our isolates expressed *fyuA* (ferric yersiniabactin uptake), a type of siderophore, which was originally detected in *Yersinia pestis*, and contributes to the pathogenicity of UPEC, especially during colonization of the urinary tract. Yersiniabactin may protect bacterial cells against the host immune response [36]. The most important ColV and ColBM virulence plasmids associated with ExPEC virulence includes the aerobactin (*iutA/iucABCD*). This operon encodes high-affinity iron-transport systems, which are used by bacteria to obtain iron in low-iron conditions such as those they encounter in host fluids and tissues. As many as 30% of our virulence-gene-associated isolates carried at least one siderophore gene, which allows these strains to survive in low iron environments, for example in the bladder or other host fluids and tissues.

Another gene found in the core genome of ExPEC large virulence plasmids is *iss*, which encodes a protein linked with increased serum survival in human *E. coli* isolates. Numerous studies have documented its strong alignment with virulent (but not with avirulent) *E. coli* strains [37]. Almost 16% of our virulence-gene-associated isolates exhibited a protection factor against phagocytosis, and moreover, connected either with adhesins or iron uptake genes and/or factors facilitating colonization.

No less important a role during infection is played by toxins, as they contribute to the spreading of bacteria in tissues, increased cytotoxicity and insensitivity to neutrophils. One of the most frequently detected genes encoding a toxin in ExPEC is *tsh* (temperature-sensitive hemagglutinin), a member of the autotransporter group of proteins first identified in avian-pathogenic *Escherichia coli* (APEC). Autotransporters are a family of autonomously secreted proteins from gram-negative bacteria exhibiting diverse functions involved in virulence, including adhesins, proteases, cytotoxins and cell invasion proteins. The above mentioned toxin contributes to the development of lesions and deposition of fibrin in avian air sacs. It can act both as an adhesin and as a serine protease, agglutinating erythrocytes while in contact with the extracellular surface of the bacterial cells. It can adhere to purified haemoglobin and bind with great efficiency to extracellular matrix proteins. It cleaves casein and exhibits mucinolytic activity [38]. This toxin was detected in 23% of our virulence-gene-associated isolates.

The important protectins/serum resistance in ExPEC involve capsula antigens *kpsII* (protection factor against phagocytosis and the spreading factor) and *cvaC* (factor facilitating colonization). In our study, we found their presence together in up to 21% of our virulence-gene-associated isolates.

E. coli strains can be classified into the following phylogenetic groups: A, B1, B2, C, D, E, F, and clade I [22]. A link between the virulence of a strain and its phylogenetic group has been previously reported by Clermont et al. [22,39]. Commensal *E. coli*, with no pathogenic features, occurring among other places on the gastrointestinal tract mucosa, most often represent group A or B1. Pathogenic *E. coli* responsible for intestinal infections represent phylogenetic groups A, B1 or D. *E. coli* responsible for extra-intestinal infections belong in groups B2 and D. Group E is related to group D (including O157: H7), while group F is related to the main group B2. Clones of *E. coli* strains, which are genetically diverse but phenotypically indistinguishable, have been assigned to cryptic clade I [40,41].

The phylogenetic grouping examined by us showed that most *E. coli* isolates belonged in groups B1 and A, followed by strains belonging in group D, while groups E and F occurred infrequently as shown in Table 2. Our results are in agreement with those reported by Rúgeles et al. and Ombarak et al. [2,42], in which *E. coli* isolated from foods mainly belonged in A and B1 phylogenetic groups. The potentially virulent strains (43 strains) were mostly classified into phylogenetic group E (100%), followed by group F (75%), group D (67%), group B1 (55%), group C (38.5%) and group A (27.6%) (Table 3).

5. Conclusions

Our obtained data suggest that *E. coli* contaminating our cheese products might have the potential for causing intestinal and, moreover, extra-intestinal infections. Although our study consists of a relatively small number of samples and therefore faces limitations in statistical analysis, it provides important information about the phylogenetic background and incidence of virulent *E. coli* isolated from cheese produced from unpasteurized ovine milk in the Slovak Republic. Our results clearly suggest that microbial quality and safety of unpasteurized cheese made from raw ovine milk produced by local farmers and distributors are not sufficiently good. The presence of coliform bacteria in raw milk products indicates not only poor hygiene, but even worse, these microorganisms are vehicles for virulent genes with the potential to cause a variety of intestinal and extra-intestinal diseases in consumers. As a relatively large number of people still consume raw milk and raw milk products, we would emphasize the increased need for food control and ensuring improved hygiene, thereby contributing to the reduction of potential public health threats.

Author Contributions: Conceptualization, D.B. and V.K.; methodology, L.K.; writing—original draft preparation, D.B. and L.K.; writing—review and editing, D.B. and L.K.; supervision, D.B. and V.K.; project administration, D.B.; funding acquisition, D.B. All authors have read and agreed to the published version of the manuscript.

Funding: This research was funded by VEGA, grant number 2/0010/21. The APC was funded by VEGA, grant number 2/0010/21.

Acknowledgments: The authors thank Martin Tomáška from Dairy Research Institute in Žilina for providing laboratory support for sample collection.

Conflicts of Interest: The authors declare no conflict of interest.

References

1. Oliver, S.P.; Jayarao, B.M.; Almeida, R.A. Foodborne Pathogens in Milk and the Dairy Farm Environment: Food Safety and Public Health Implications. *Foodborne Pathog. Dis.* **2005**, *2*, 115–129. [CrossRef] [PubMed]
2. Ombarak, R.; Hinenoya, A.; Awasthi, S.P.; Iguchi, A.; Shima, A.; Elbagory, A.; Yamasaki, S. Prevalence and pathogenic potential of Escherichia coli isolates from raw milk and raw milk cheese in Egypt. *Int. J. Food Microbiol.* **2016**, *221*, 69–76. [CrossRef] [PubMed]

3. Yoon, Y.; Lee, S.; Choi, K.-H. Microbial benefits and risks of raw milk cheese. *Food Control* **2016**, *63*, 201–215. [CrossRef]
4. Ioanna, F.; Quaglia, N.C.; Storelli, M.; Castiglia, D.; Goffredo, E.; Storelli, A.; De Rosa, M.; Normanno, G.; Jambrenghi, A.C.; Dambrosio, A. Survival of Escherichia coli O157:H7 during the manufacture and ripening of Cacioricotta goat cheese. *Food Microbiol.* **2018**, *70*, 200–205. [CrossRef] [PubMed]
5. Cancino-Padilla, N.; De Chile, P.U.C.; Fellenberg, M.A.; Franco, W.; Ibáñez, R.A.; Vargas-Bello-Pérez, E. Foodborne bacteria in dairy products: Detection by molecular techniques. *Cienc. E Investig. Agrar.* **2017**, *44*, 215–229. [CrossRef]
6. Gill, A.; Oudit, D.; Alexander, P. Enumeration of Escherichia coli O157 in Outbreak-Associated Gouda Cheese Made with Raw Milk. *J. Food Prot.* **2015**, *78*, 1733–1737. [CrossRef]
7. Mccollum, J.T.; Williams, N.J.; Beam, S.W.; Cosgrove, S.; Ettestad, P.J.; Ghosh, T.S.; Kimura, A.C.; Nguyen, L.; Stroika, S.G.; Vogt, R.L.; et al. Multistate Outbreak of Escherichia coli O157:H7 Infections Associated with In-Store Sampling of an Aged Raw-Milk Gouda Cheese, 2010. *J. Food Prot.* **2012**, *75*, 1759–1765. [CrossRef]
8. Kaper, J.B.; Nataro, J.P.; Mobley, H. Pathogenic Escherichia coli. *Nat. Rev. Genet.* **2004**, *2*, 123–140. [CrossRef]
9. Bielaszewska, M.; Mellmann, A.; Zhang, W.; Köck, R.; Fruth, A.; Bauwens, A.; Peters, G.; Karch, H. Characterisation of the Escherichia coli strain associated with an outbreak of haemolytic uraemic syndrome in Germany, 2011: A microbiological study. *Lancet Infect. Dis.* **2011**, *11*, 671–676. [CrossRef]
10. Dallman, T.; Cross, L.; Bishop, P.; Perry, N.; Olesen, B.; Grant, K.A.; Jenkins, C. Whole Genome Sequencing of an Unusual Serotype of Shiga Toxin–producingEscherichia coli. *Emerg. Infect. Dis.* **2013**, *19*, 1302–1304. [CrossRef]
11. Brussow, H.; Canchaya, C.; Hardt, W.-D. Phages and the Evolution of Bacterial Pathogens: From Genomic Rearrangements to Lysogenic Conversion. *Microbiol. Mol. Biol. Rev.* **2004**, *68*, 560–602. [CrossRef]
12. Costanzo, N.; Ceniti, C.; Santoro, A.; Clausi, M.T.; Casalinuovo, F. Foodborne Pathogen Assessment in Raw Milk Cheeses. *Int. J. Food Sci.* **2020**, *2020*, 3616713. [CrossRef]
13. O'Loughin, E. Escherichia coli O157:H7. *Lancet* **1997**, *349*, 1553. [CrossRef]
14. European Food Safety Authority and European Centre for Disease Prevention and Control (EFSA and ECDC). The European Union summary report on trends and sources of zoonoses, zoonotic agents and food-borne outbreaks in 2017. *EFSA J.* **2018**, *16*, e05500. [CrossRef]
15. Aslam, M.; Toufeer, M.; Bravo, C.N.; Lai, V.; Rempel, H.; Manges, A.; Diarra, M.S. Characterization of Extraintestinal Pathogenic Escherichia coli isolated from retail poultry meats from Alberta, Canada. *Int. J. Food Microbiol.* **2014**, *177*, 49–56. [CrossRef]
16. Nordstrom, L.; Liu, C.M.; Price, L.B. Foodborne urinary tract infections: A new paradigm for antimicrobial-resistant foodborne illness. *Front. Microbiol.* **2013**, *4*, 29. [CrossRef] [PubMed]
17. Johnson, J.R.; Russo, T.A. Extraintestinal pathogenic Escherichia coli: "The other bad *E. coli*". *J. Lab. Clin. Med.* **2002**, *139*, 155–162. [CrossRef] [PubMed]
18. Singer, R.S. Urinary tract infections attributed to diverse ExPEC strains in food animals: Evidence and data gaps. *Front. Microbiol.* **2015**, *6*, 28. [CrossRef] [PubMed]
19. Altalhi, A.D.; Hassan, S. Bacterial quality of raw milk investigated by Escherichia coli and isolates analysis for specific virulence-gene markers. *Food Control* **2009**, *20*, 913–917. [CrossRef]
20. Paneto, B.; Schocken-Iturrino, R.; Macedo, C.; Santo, E.; Marin, J. Occurrence of toxigenic Escherichia coli in raw milk cheese in Brazil. *Arq. Bras. Med. Vet. Zootec.* **2007**, *59*, 508–512. [CrossRef]
21. Bessède, E.; Angla-Gre, M.; Delagarde, Y.; Hieng, S.S.; Menard, A.; Mégraud, F. Matrix-Assisted laser-desorption/ionization BIOTYPER: Experience in the routine of a University hospital. *Clin. Microbiol. Infect.* **2011**, *17*, 533–538. [CrossRef] [PubMed]
22. Clermont, O.; Christenson, J.K.; Denamur, E.; Gordon, D.M. The ClermontEscherichia coliphylo-typing method revisited: Improvement of specificity and detection of new phylo-groups. *Environ. Microbiol. Rep.* **2012**, *5*, 58–65. [CrossRef] [PubMed]
23. Lescat, M.; Clermont, O.; Woerther, P.L.; Glodt, J.; Dion, S.; Skurnik, D.; Djossou, F.; Dupont, C.; Perroz, G.; Picard, B.; et al. CommensalEscherichia colistrains in Guiana reveal a high genetic diversity with host-dependant population structure. *Environ. Microbiol. Rep.* **2012**, *5*, 49–57. [CrossRef] [PubMed]
24. Johnson, J.R.; Stell, A. Extended Virulence Genotypes of *Escherichia coli* Strains from Patients with Urosepsis in Relation to Phylogeny and Host Compromise. *J. Infect. Dis.* **2000**, *181*, 261–272. [CrossRef] [PubMed]
25. Ewers, C.; Kießling, S.; Wilking, H.; Kiebling, S.; Alt, K.; Antáo, E.-M.; Laturnus, C.; Diehl, I.; Glodde, S.; Homeier, T. Avian pathogenic, uropathogenic, and newborn meningitis-causing Escherichia coli: How closely related are they? *Int. J. Med. Microbiol.* **2007**, *297*, 163–176. [CrossRef] [PubMed]
26. Le Bouguenec, C.; Archambaud, M.; Labigne, A. Rapid and specific detection of the pap, afa, and sfa adhesin-encoding operons in uropathogenic Escherichia coli strains by polymerase chain reaction. *J. Clin. Microbiol.* **1992**, *30*, 1189–1193. [CrossRef] [PubMed]
27. Dozois, C.M.; Dho-Moulin, M.; Brée, A.; Fairbrother, J.M.; Desautels, C.; Curtiss, R. Relationship between the Tsh Autotransporter and Pathogenicity of Avian Escherichia coli and Localization and Analysis of the tsh Genetic Region. *Infect. Immun.* **2000**, *68*, 4145–4154. [CrossRef]
28. Pass, M.A.; Odedra, R.; Batt, R.M. Multiplex PCRs for Identification of Escherichia coli Virulence Genes. *J. Clin. Microbiol.* **2000**, *38*, 2001–2004. [CrossRef]
29. Holko, I.; Bisova, T.; Holkova, Z.; Kmet, V. Virulence markers of Escherichia coli strains isolated from traditional cheeses made from unpasteurised sheep milk in Slovakia. *Food Control* **2006**, *17*, 393–396. [CrossRef]

30. Skočková, A.; Koláčková, I.; Kubelová, M.; Karpíšková, R. Shiga toxin-producing Escherichia coli (STEC) in the Czech Re-public: Characterization of pathogenic strains isolated from pig and cattle carcasses. *J. Food Nutr. Res.* **2017**, *56*, 362–371.
31. Friedrich, A.W.; Bielaszewska, M.; Zhang, W.; Pulz, M.; Kuczius, T.; Ammon, A.; Karch, H. Escherichia coli Harboring Shiga Toxin 2 Gene Variants: Frequency and Association with Clinical Symptoms. *J. Infect. Dis.* **2002**, *185*, 74–84. [CrossRef] [PubMed]
32. Panel, E.B.; Koutsoumanis, K.; Allende, A.; Alvarez-Ordóñez, A.; Bover-Cid, S.; Chemaly, M.; Davies, R.; De Cesare, A.; Herman, L.; Hilbert, F.; et al. Pathogenicity assessment of Shiga toxin-producing Escherichia coli (STEC) and the public health risk posed by contamination of food with STEC. *EFSA J.* **2020**, *18*. [CrossRef]
33. Morabito, S. *Pathogenic Escherichia Coli: Molecular and Cellular Microbiology*; Caister Academic Press: Norfolk, VA, USA, 2014; ISBN 9781908230379.
34. Farrokh, C.; Jordan, K.; Auvray, F.; Glass, K.; Oppegaard, H.; Raynaud, S.; Thevenot, D.; Condron, R.; De Reu, K.; Govaris, A.; et al. Review of Shiga-toxin-producing Escherichia coli (STEC) and their significance in dairy production. *Int. J. Food Microbiol.* **2013**, *162*, 190–212. [CrossRef]
35. Guzman-Hernandez, R.; Contreras-Rodriguez, A.; Hernandez-Velez, R.; Perez-Martinez, I.; Lopez-Merino, A.; Zaidi, M.B.; Estrada-Garcia, T. Mexican unpasteurised fresh cheeses are contaminated with Salmonella spp., non-O157 Shiga toxin producing Escherichia coli and potential uropathogenic E. coli strains: A public health risk. *Int. J. Food Microbiol.* **2016**, *237*, 10–16. [CrossRef] [PubMed]
36. Garénaux, A.; Caza, M.; Dozois, C.M. The Ins and Outs of siderophore mediated iron uptake by extra-intestinal pathogenic Escherichia coli. *Veter. Microbiol.* **2011**, *153*, 89–98. [CrossRef]
37. Sarowska, J.; Futoma-Kołoch, B.; Jama-Kmiecik, A.; Frej-Madrzak, M.; Ksiazczyk, M.; Bugla-Ploskonska, G.; Choroszy-Krol, I. Virulence factors, prevalence and potential transmission of extraintestinal pathogenic Escherichia coli isolated from different sources: Recent reports. *Gut Pathog.* **2019**, *11*, 1–16. [CrossRef]
38. Kostakioti, M.; Stathopoulos, C. Functional Analysis of the Tsh Autotransporter from an Avian Pathogenic Escherichia coli Strain. *Infect. Immun.* **2004**, *72*, 5548–5554. [CrossRef]
39. Clermont, O.; Bonacorsi, S.; Bingen, E. Rapid and Simple Determination of the Escherichia coli Phylogenetic Group. *Appl. Environ. Microbiol.* **2000**, *66*, 4555–4558. [CrossRef]
40. Köhler, C.-D.; Dobrindt, U. What defines extraintestinal pathogenic Escherichia coli? *Int. J. Med. Microbiol.* **2011**, *301*, 642–647. [CrossRef]
41. Tivendale, K.; Logue, C.M.; Kariyawasam, S.; Jordan, D.; Hussein, A.; Li, G.; Wannemuehler, Y.; Nolan, L.K. Avian-Pathogenic Escherichia coli Strains Are Similar to Neonatal Meningitis *E. coli* Strains and Are Able To Cause Meningitis in the Rat Model of Human Disease. *Infect. Immun.* **2010**, *78*, 3412–3419. [CrossRef]
42. Rúgeles, L.C.; Bai, J.; Martínez, A.J.; Vanegas, M.C.; Gómez-Duarte, O.G. Molecular characterization of diarrheagenic Escherichia coli strains from stools samples and food products in Colombia. *Int. J. Food Microbiol.* **2010**, *138*, 282–286. [CrossRef] [PubMed]

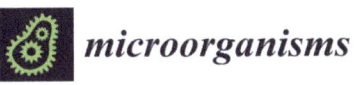

Article

Successful Dissemination of Plasmid-Mediated Extended-Spectrum β-Lactamases in Enterobacterales over Humans to Wild Fauna

Racha Beyrouthy [1,2], Carolina Sabença [3,4,5], Frédéric Robin [1,2], Patricia Poeta [3,6], Giberto Igrejas [4,5,6] and Richard Bonnet [1,2,*]

1. Institut National de la Santé et de la Recherche Médicale, (UMR1071), Institut National de la Recherche Agronomique (USC-2018), Université Clermont Auvergne, 63000 Clermont-Ferrand, France; rbeyrouthy@chu-clermontferrand.fr (R.B.); frobin@chu-clermontferrand.fr (F.R.)
2. Centre National de Référence de la Résistance aux Antibiotiques, Centre Hospitalier Universitaire, 63000 Clermont-Ferrand, France
3. MicroART-Antibiotic Resistance Team, Department of Veterinary Sciences, University of Trá-os-Montes and Alto Douro (UTAD), 5001-801 Vila Real, Portugal; carolinasabenca@hotmail.com (C.S.); ppoeta@utad.pt (P.P.)
4. Department of Genetics and Biotechnology, University of Trás-os-Montes and Alto Douro, 5001-801 Vila Real, Portugal; gigrejas@utad.pt
5. Functional Genomics and Proteomics Unit, University of Trás-os-Montes and Alto Douro, 5001-801 Vila Real, Portugal
6. Associated Laboratory for Green Chemistry (LAQV-REQUIMTE), University NOVA of Lisbon, 2825-168 Caparica, Portugal
* Correspondence: rbonnet@chu-clermontferrand.fr; Tel.: +33-473754920

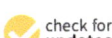

Citation: Beyrouthy, R.; Sabença, C.; Robin, F.; Poeta, P.; Igrejas, G.; Bonnet, R. Successful Dissemination of Plasmid-Mediated Extended-Spectrum β-Lactamases in Enterobacterales over Humans to Wild Fauna. *Microorganisms* 2021, 9, 1471. https://doi.org/10.3390/microorganisms9071471

Academic Editors: Dobroslava Bujňáková, Nikola Puvača and Ivana Ćirković

Received: 22 June 2021
Accepted: 7 July 2021
Published: 9 July 2021

Publisher's Note: MDPI stays neutral with regard to jurisdictional claims in published maps and institutional affiliations.

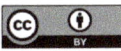

Copyright: © 2021 by the authors. Licensee MDPI, Basel, Switzerland. This article is an open access article distributed under the terms and conditions of the Creative Commons Attribution (CC BY) license (https://creativecommons.org/licenses/by/4.0/).

Abstract: Background: The emergence of multidrug-resistant bacteria remains poorly understood in the wild ecosystem and at the interface of habitats. Here, we explored the spread of *Escherichia coli* containing IncI1-ST3 plasmid encoding resistance gene *cefotaximase-Munich-1* ($bla_{CTX-M-1}$) in human-influenced habitats and wild fauna using a genomic approach. Methods. Multilocus sequence typing (MLST), single-nucleotide polymorphism comparison, synteny-based analysis and data mining approaches were used to analyse a dataset of genomes and circularised plasmids. Results. CTX-M-1 *E. coli* sequence types (STs) were preferentially associated with ecosystems. Few STs were shared by distinct habitats. IncI1-ST3-$bla_{CTX-M-1}$ plasmids are disseminated among all *E. coli* phylogroups. The main divergences in plasmids were located in a shuffling zone including $bla_{CTX-M-1}$ inserted in a conserved site. This insertion hot spot exhibited diverse positions and orientations in a zone-modulating conjugation, and the resulting synteny was associated with geographic and biological sources. Conclusions. The ecological success of IncI1-ST3-$bla_{CTX-M-1}$ appears less linked to the spread of their bacterial recipients than to their ability to transfer in a broad spectrum of bacterial lineages. This feature is associated with the diversity of their shuffling conjugation region that contain $bla_{CTX-M-1}$. These might be involved in the resistance to antimicrobials, but also in their spread.

Keywords: *Escherichia coli*; β-lactamase; plasmid; CTX-M-1; IncI1-ST3

1. Introduction

In recent decades, the consumption of antimicrobials has been rising in both humans and animals, and as a result, so has the prevalence of plasmid-mediated extended-spectrum β-lactamases (ESBLs) [1]. However, ESBLs confer resistance to penicillins and cephalosporins, including last-generation cephalosporins, which are key molecules for treating infections caused by Gram-negative bacteria in hospitals [1]. Consequently, the last-generation cephalosporins are classified by the World Health Organization (WHO) as critically important antimicrobial agents in human medicine [2]. The ESBLs are inhibited by clavulanic acid, sulbactam and tazobactam, and they are not efficient against carbapenem antimicrobials. Their main reservoir is Enterobacterales, especially the widespread and versatile species *Escherichia coli*, which is one of the intestinal microbiota and a major pathogen in humans and animals.

Antimicrobial resistance (AMR) is a complex and multifaceted threat to humans, animals, and the environment. A major cause of the AMR burden is the capability of resistant bacteria such as *E. coli* and AMR-encoding genes to spread between individuals, including across sectors by horizontal gene transfer. Plasmids are extra-chromosomal mobile genetic elements that play an essential role in bacterial ecology and evolution and they help their hosts adapt to a multitude of environments [3]. Plasmids carry accessory genes, including most clinically relevant resistance genes, such as those encoding carbapenemases [4], cephalosporinases [5] and the widespread ESBLs [6–8] that can spread across high-risk bacterial clones [9,10]. The most frequently detected ESBLs are class A β-lactamases. They represented by three major types: cefotaximase-Munich (CTX-M), temoneira (TEM) and sulfhydryl variable (SHV) and they include more than 400 variants reported today. These corresponding genes are often associated with other genes that confer resistance to beta-lactams and other antimicrobial agents such as quinolones, aminoglycosides and sulfonamides [7,8].

Initially, ESBLs were variants of TEM- and SHV-type penicillinases that acquired hydrolytic activity against oxyimino cephalosporins, also called third- and fourth-generation cephalosporins (C3G/C4G) through 1- to 4-point mutations. These enzymes were mainly observed during the 1980s and the 1990s in nosocomial Enterobacterales, such as *Klebsiella pneumoniae* and *Enterobacter cloacae*, which are mainly responsible for infections in immunocompromised patients in intensive care units [6–8]. Since the early 2000s, CTX-M-type ESBLs have been the dominant ESBLs all over the world, owing to their strong association with the species *E. coli*. This recipient, which is a major pathobiont of the mammal gut, favours the spread not only in intensive care units, as observed for TEM- and SHV-type ESBLs, but also in all other care units of hospitals and the community [5–7]. Consequently, the CTX-M-type ESBLs, especially variants CTX-M-15 and CTX-M-1, are community-acquired ESBLs, which have almost substituted for the TEM- and SHV-type ESBLs, and they are the most common plasmid-mediated ESBL among Enterobacterales isolates of human and veterinary origin worldwide [11–15]. CTX-M-15 is encoded by genes located in IncF plasmids harboured by *E. coli* ST131 clade C, a clade strongly associated with human hosts. CTX-M-1 is observed in *E. coli* strains collected from humans and animals, and its gene $bla_{CTX-M-1}$ has been associated mainly with the broad host range IncN plasmids, and much more frequently in the narrow host range IncI1 [16–25].

The IncI plasmids belong to the I-complex plasmid family including the incompatibility groups IncI1, IncIγ, IncB, IncZ and IncK [26]. The IncI1 plasmid backbone is organised into four major conserved regions encoding replication, conjugative transfer, stability and leading [27,28], in addition to variable regions encoding accessory functions such as antimicrobial gene resistance.

There is a great concern that contacts with animals may enhance the risk of acquiring ESBL-encoding plasmids by humans [29,30]. IncI1-ST3 plasmids are one of the most prevalent plasmids in ESBL CTX-M-1 in Enterobacterales isolated from humans, animals and environmental sources [18–25]. However, the relationships at the interface of humans and animals remain elusive, especially for wild animals. This study compared CTX-M-1-producing *E. coli* isolates and IncI1-ST3 plasmids collected from humans, food-producing animals, and wild animals to best understand the CTX-M-1 spread among these ecosystems.

2. Materials and Methods

Genomic dataset. For this study, we collected 122 *E. coli* whole genome sequences (WGSs) containing IncI1-ST3 plasmids and $bla_{CTX-M-1}$ (Supplementary Tables S1 and S2). The dataset includes WGSs sequenced during this study ($n = 43$) and recovered from GenBank ($n = 79$) after filtering for quality (ATCG assembly size >4.5 Mb, contigs number <200 and N50 > 60,000) and the availability of metadata. The sources of strains were humans ($n = 57$), domestic animals ($n = 11$), food or food-producing animals ($n = 37$), wild animals

(n = 13) [20,31–37] and municipal wastewater (n = 1). Three strains were from unknown origins. Of this collection, 30 human strains and 13 strains isolated from wild animals were sequenced for this study (Supplementary Table S1). The other data were collected from the NCBI Short Read Archive (SRA) or the European Nucleotide Archive (ENA) by screening of the *E. coli* genomes of the GenBank database (Supplementary Table S2). The screening for encoding CTX-M-1- and IncI1-ST3-specific alleles was performed with DIAMOND and blastn software, respectively, using 100% identity threshold and 100% coverage threshold.

Likewise, 20,668 non-redundant complete plasmids collected from GenBank were screened for the IncI1-ST3 feature and the presence of $bla_{CTX-M-1}$. It resulted in a collection of 39 IncI1-ST3-$bla_{CTX-M-1}$ circularised plasmids (Supplementary Table S3).

Whole genome sequencing (WGS). This was performed using the next-generation sequencing platform of the teaching hospital of Clermont-Ferrand, France. DNA was extracted with a DNeasy UltraClean Microbial kit (Qiagen, Hilden, Germany). The libraries were prepared with a Nextera XT Kit (Illumina, San Diego, CA, USA), and they were sequenced by the Illumina MiSeq system, generating 2 × 301-base pair (bp) paired-end reads. Fastp software v0.19.10 [38] was used for quality filtering of Illumina reads, and SPAdes was used for short reads assembly [39]. The mean sequencing depth was $\geq 163\times$; the number of assembled contigs ranged between 51 and 175, the mean contig number was 99.77, the N50 ranged between 63,075 and 383,707, and the mean contig number was 186,502. The genome sizes ranged between 4,667,864 and 5,338,201 nucleotides. The raw reads have been deposited in the European Nucleotide Archive (ENA, https://www.ebi.ac.uk/ena) under project accession number PRJEB36175.

Molecular typing. *E. coli* phylogroups and multilocus sequence typing (MLST) were determined in silico according to the Clermont Typing method [40] and Achtman's MLST scheme [41]. The molecular typing of isolates was performed by core genome SNP-based typing (cgSNP). BactSNP was used to perform cgSNP using the *E. coli* core genome downloaded from the Enterobase website (https://enterobase.warwick.ac.uk) as a reference, as previously described [42,43]. After the filtration of recombination zones detected by Gubbins [44], a phylogenetic tree was inferred from the resulting alignment by maximum likelihood using RAxML [45].

Antimicrobial gene detection. The antimicrobial-resistant genes were identified by alignment against a database including the online databases CARD [46], Resfinder [47], and the NCBI National Database of Antibiotic Resistant Organisms (https://www.ncbi.nlm.nih.gov/pathogens/antimicrobial-resistance/ (accessed on 1 April 2021)) using a 95% minimum threshold for the breadth of coverage and identity percentage, as previously described [48].

Synteny analysis. This was performed with the Sibelia package [49]. The presence/absence matrix inferring from the resulting synteny blocks was analysed by multiple correspondence analysis (MCA) and hierarchical clustering (HC) in R with package FactoMiner (https://www.r-project.org).

3. Results

3.1. Whole Genome Typing of E. coli Harbouring Plasmids IncI1-ST3 and $bla_{CTX-M-1}$

To best understand the large diffusion of the CTX-M-1 ESBL, we collected a dataset comprising 122 *E. coli* WGSs containing IncI1-ST3 replicon and $bla_{CTX-M-1}$ isolated from humans, human-influenced habitats and wild fauna. The corresponding genomes were classified into eight major phylogenetic branches by SNP-based core genome typing. These major branches corresponded to the *E. coli* phylogroups (Figure 1).

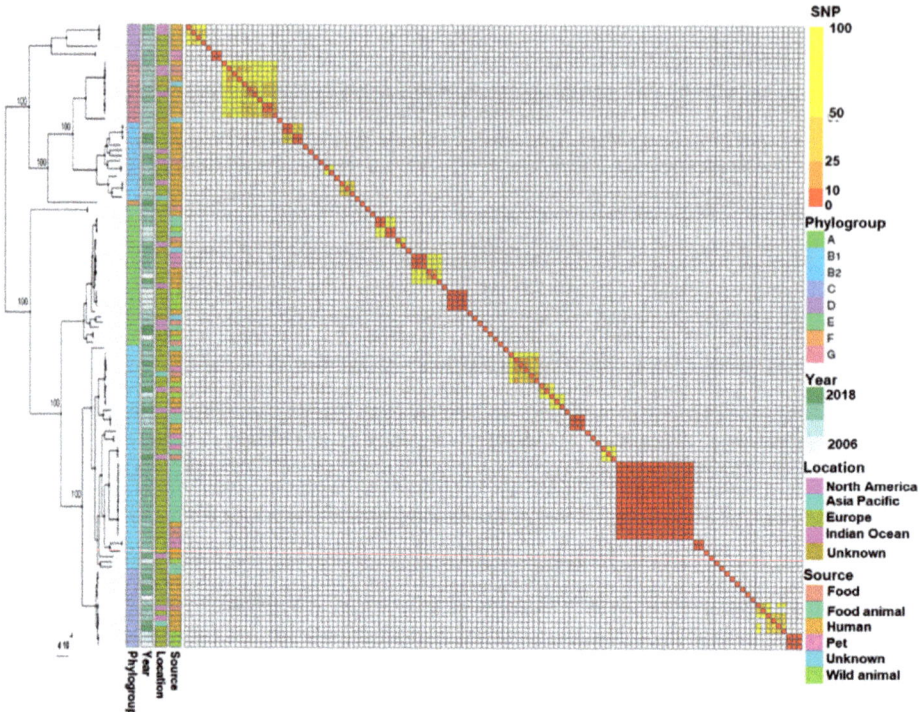

Figure 1. Phylogenetic tree and corresponding distance matrix based on SNPs of *E. coli* WGSs containing plasmids IncI1-ST3 encoding $bla_{CTX-M-1}$. SNP calling, SNP filtering and tree inferring were performed with bactSNP, Gubbins and RAxML, respectively. The bootstrap values are indicated for the major phylogenetic branches as percentages for 500 replications.

Most genomes belonged to phylogroups B1 (35.8%, n = 43), A (20.8%, n = 25), B2 (12.5%, n = 15), C (12.5%, n = 15) and G (10%, n = 12). The distribution of genomes among the phylogroups significantly differed depending on the originating source (Fisher test, p-value < 0.001). Since the genomes of phylogroups A and B1 frequently originated from food or food-producing animals (50% and 67%, respectively), the B2 genomes preferentially originated from humans (93.3% versus 6.7% from food and food-producing animals).

Human *E. coli* strains (n = 51/57) were distantly related, except for three clusters of two strains diverging by ≤10 SNPs and belonging to ST117 (n = 2) and ST12 (n = 2 × 2). The clonal isolates (divergence ≤ 10 SNPs) mainly clustered isolates from food and animals including wild animals. Few clonal clusters and STs contained isolates from different habitats (Figure 2), with possible cross-transmissions between humans and human-influenced habitats, and between wild and food-producing animals.

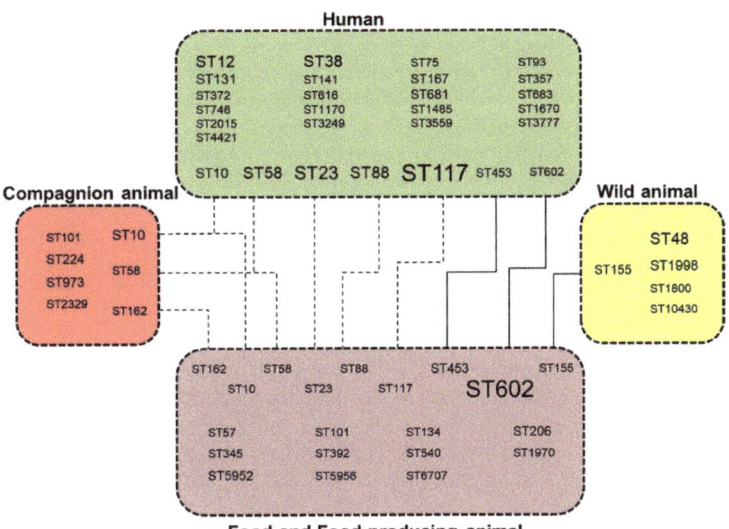

Figure 2. Distribution of *E. coli* ST lineages in human, human-influenced habitats and wild fauna showing deduced transmission pathways between these ecosystems. Dashed lines indicate STs shared by different habitats, and solid lines indicate closely related isolates diverging by ≤10 SNPs.

3.2. Antimicrobial Resistance Genes

In addition to the chromosome-mediated ampC gene encoding cephalosporinase, 45 acquired antimicrobial resistance mechanisms were associated with $bla_{CTX-M-1}$ (Figure 3). None of the genes were strictly conserved.

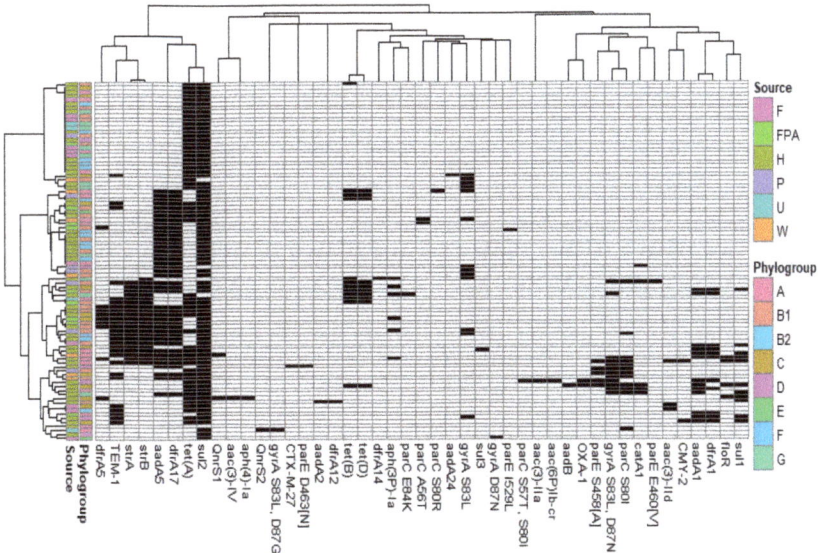

Figure 3. Antimicrobial resistance mechanisms associated with non-redundant *E. coli* harbouring $bla_{CTX-M-1}$ and IncI1-ST3 plasmids (black: presence; white: absence). Source: F, food; FPA, food-producing animals; H, human; P, pet; U: unknown and W, wild animal.

Excluding the redundant isolates corresponding to clonal isolates ($n = 30$), the most frequent genes were sulphonamide resistance gene *sul2* (94.4%), tetracycline resistance gene *tet(A)* (63.3%), streptomycin/spectinomycin resistance genes *aadA5* (47.8%), *strB* (24.4%) and *strA* (23.3%), trimethoprim resistance gene *dfrA17* (47.8%), and penicillinase-encoding gene *bla*$_{TEM-1}$ (30.0%) (Supplementary Figure S1a). The investigation of resistance gene co-occurrence revealed preferential associations. Among the most frequent genes, *aadA5*, *dfrA17*, *strA*, *strB* and *bla*$_{TEM-1}$ exhibited a strong association index. This suggests their frequent coexistence with *bla*$_{CTX-M-1}$ probably in the same plasmid IncI1-ST3 (Supplementary Figure S1b).

3.3. SNP Analysis of bla$_{CTX-M-1}$-Encoding Plasmids IncI1-ST3

A total of 117 assemblies (96%) contained a contig harbouring *bla*$_{CTX-M-1}$, IS*Ecp1* and at least the B segment of a region previously called shufflon that is specific to IncI1 plasmids [50]. The well-known mobile block IS*Ecp1*-*bla*$_{CTX-M-1}$ [51,52] was located 333 pb upstream of the B segment of the shufflon. In four cases, mobile element IS*Kpn26* was inserted between *bla*$_{CTX-M-1}$ and IS*Ecp1*. The *bla*$_{CTX-M-1}$ gene was encoded by plasmids IncI1 in most *E. coli* harbouring this family of plasmids. SNP analysis of IncI1-ST3 plasmids encoding *bla*$_{CTX-M-1}$ showed that they differ by <10 SNPs and most often by 1–2 SNPs. The resulting tree had a comb-like shape constituting a unique major clade (Figure 4).

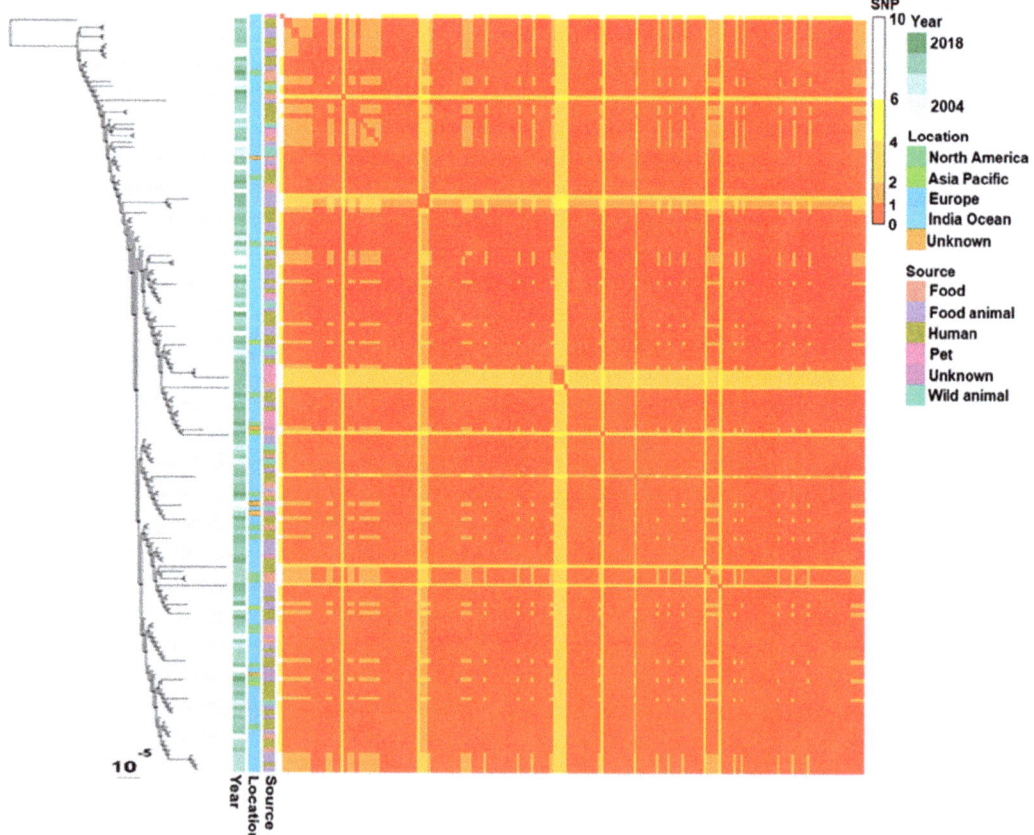

Figure 4. Phylogenetic tree and corresponding distance matrix based on SNPs of plasmids IncI1-ST3 encoding *bla*$_{CTX-M-1}$. SNP calling, SNP filtering and tree inferring were performed with bactSNP, Gubbins and RAxML, respectively.

3.4. Synteny Variation in $bla_{CTX-M-1}$-Encoding Plasmids IncI1-ST3

Although not explored for epidemiologic investigations, genetic rearrangements are a major driving force of plasmid evolution. Therefore, we investigated synteny variations in 39 circularised IncI1-ST3-$bla_{CTX-M-1}$ plasmids. The synteny analysis by multiple correspondence analysis (MCA) and hierarchical clustering (HC) classified the plasmids into six major clusters (Figure 5). The clusters are supported by statistical tests (Adonis test's p-value: 0.001 and R^2: 0.75; Dispersion permutation test's p-value: 0.1).

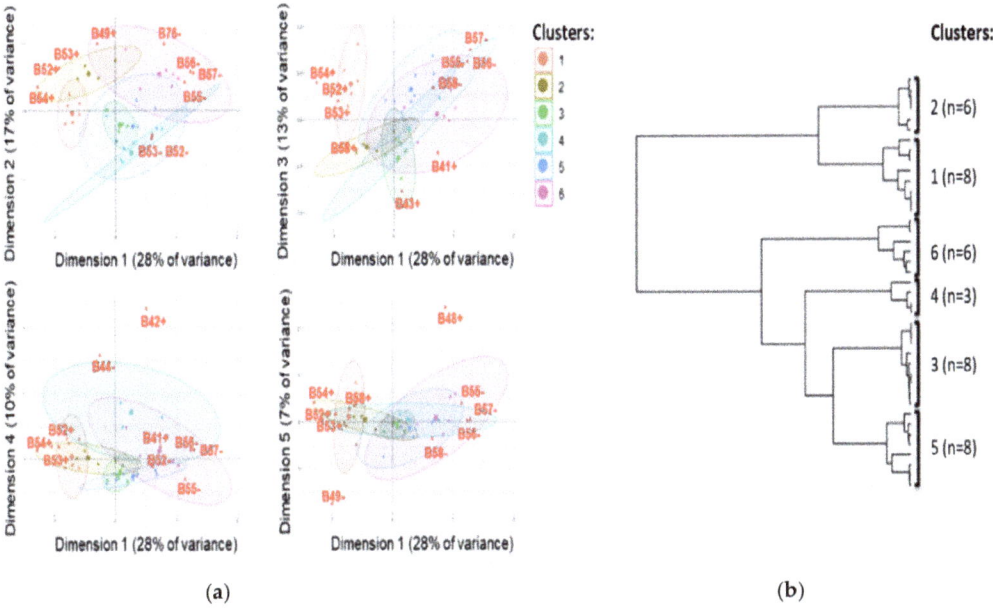

Figure 5. Multiple corresponding analysis (**a**) and hierarchical clustering (**b**) inferring synteny analysis of 39 circularised plasmids IncI1-ST3 encoding $bla_{CTX-M-1}$. The clusters are surrounded by 95% confidence ellipses, and the 10 most contributory synteny blocks of sequences are indicated in red (B#: shuffling segment B associated with IS*Ecp1* and $bla_{CTX-M-1}$; #: position of the genetic feature, rv: reverse and fd: forward).

Among the 14 synteny blocks that were significantly associated with the clusters (FDR-adjusted X2-test's p-values, 1.4×10^{-6} to 5.5×10^{-3}), 13 were in the unique shufflon region between the conserved genes *rci* and *pilV*. The genetic features in region *rci-pilV* are specific to IncI1 plasmids, and they comprise up to four DNA segments A to D, previously identified as randomly rearranged by recombinase Rci [50]. This region harboured the most synteny variations.

The synteny of *rci-pilV* was also investigated from *E. coli* WGSs. A total of 77 WGS-encoding plasmids IncI1-ST3 exhibited a complete shufflon assembly, including $bla_{CTX-M-1}$. MCA and HC analyses of synteny variants from WGSs confirmed the classification of plasmids in six major clusters (Supplementary Figures S2–S4). Segment D was absent in all plasmids, and mobile element IS*Ecp1*-$bla_{CTX-M-1}$ was always located downstream from segment B to form a conserved block exhibiting different positions in the shufflon. This block can affect the shuffling process, and it was paradoxically the feature that contributed most to diversity (Supplementary Figure S2). The shufflon segments are involved in the synthesis of PilV adhesins of the conjugative pilus [53]. Therefore, the shuffling of segments associated with IS*Ecp1*-$bla_{CTX-M-1}$ insertion generates diversity in the PilV-encoding region.

This can modulate the recognition of recipient cells during IncI1-ST3-$bla_{\text{CTX-M-1}}$ conjugation and therefore probably their dissemination.

At the highest level of classification resolution, synteny analysis revealed 16 clusters of two to seven plasmids sharing identical synteny (Supplementary Figures S3 and S4). Ten of these clusters included plasmids isolated from the same country and the same source. Seven clusters were specific to the source. Nine clusters were only observed in human-influenced habitats. The plasmids isolated from wild animals were included in four clusters; two were specific to wild fauna, and the two others supported a possible spread between human-influenced animals and wild fauna.

4. Discussion

The increase in antimicrobial resistance worldwide is a result of inappropriate use of antimicrobials during the last decades, including those used for human medication and animal husbandry. This broad use increases the selective pressure on both commensal and pathogenic bacteria, which can spread between different ecosystems [1,54]. Livestock animals may act as reservoirs of AMR and multidrug resistant bacteria. This can lead to dissemination of AMR into humans directly by contact and the food chain or indirectly from the environment [1,54].

In this study, we analysed genomic data belonging to *E. coli* isolates collected from humans, animals (food-producing animals, companion animals, wildlife), and food samples to understand the interaction between these ecosystems in the diffusion of IncI1-ST3 plasmids encoding $bla_{\text{CTX-M-1}}$. The genomic data analysis showed that the *E. coli* phylogroups harbouring IncI1-ST3 plasmids encoding $bla_{\text{CTX-M-1}}$ significantly differed depending on the originating source. Of the isolates, 68% belonged to the phylogenetic A, B1 and C, which are associated with multiple antimicrobial resistance genes especially those encoding sulphonamide and tetracycline resistance. MLST revealed 50 sequence types. The most abundant sequence type was ST602, followed by ST117 and ST10. The correlation between ST602, which was the most abundant sequence type detected in *E. coli* phylogenetic group B1 isolates in this study, and food-producing animals was pointed out in recent reports [55–57].

Human contamination by ESBL-producing Enterobacterales from animals is often supposed, and food is considered a direct transmission vehicle. ESBL gene $bla_{\text{CTX-M-1}}$ and IncI1-ST3 plasmids were widespread in humans, human-influenced habitats and wild fauna, as previously observed [21–25]. Here, we observed that IncI1-ST3-$bla_{\text{CTX-M-1}}$ plasmids also have disseminated into all *E. coli* lineages, which cover a broad diversity of bacteria and different lifestyles, including commensal and pathogenic strains. Few clonal clusters and STs were shared by different habitats, suggesting *E. coli* lineages have a preferential habitat and few of them are involved in cross-sector spread. As shuttles, these subgroups may be risk factors for spreading antimicrobial resistance and they might be preferential targets for strategies to prevent the spread of antimicrobial resistance.

The SNP-based comparison of $bla_{\text{CTX-M-1}}$ IncI1-ST3 plasmids originating from several continents revealed a core genome highly conserved. This suggests that the dissemination of these plasmids across all sources over distant areas took decades. However, the evolutionary rate of bacterial genomes may not generate enough variations to resolve recent epidemiological processes involving small genetic elements such as IncI1-ST3-$bla_{\text{CTX-M-1}}$ plasmids. Recombination, gain and loss of DNA fragments are key processes of evolution [58]. They affect synteny and are not investigated by comparisons based on core genome SNPs. The analysis of synteny in complete $bla_{\text{CTX-M-1}}$ IncI1-ST3 plasmids revealed more diversity than SNP analysis. Synteny-based clusters were associated with sampling sources and geographic origins. This suggests that synteny analysis can be a useful approach for monitoring IncI1-ST3 plasmid spread over short periods, and it might help to analyse transmission chains.

Most variations in synteny were observed in a single region, which was previously designated shufflon and encoding a recombinase and targeted DNA segments [50]. Most diversity resulted from the positioning and orientation of a conserved block including the shufflon segment B, IS*Ecp1* and *bla*$_{CTX-M-1}$. Shufflon B appears, therefore, as a hot spot for the insertion of mobile element IS*Ecp1* and associated gene *bla*$_{CTX-M-1}$. Since IS*Ecp1* is involved in the mobilisation of ESBL- and cephalosporinase-encoding genes [51,59], shufflon B of IncI1 explains the key role of these plasmids in the spread of resistance to last-generation cephalosporins.

The assembly of *bla*$_{CTX-M-1}$ from short reads suggest a certain stability and/or the preponderance of a shufflon synteny within a bacterial clone. This contrasts with plasmids IncI2 harbouring active shufflons [60]. This stability was confirmed by assembly from long-read sequencing, which did not reveal alternative conformation of shufflons [61] and may be explained by the insertion of IS*Ecp1*-*bla*$_{CTX-M-1}$ in the shuffling zone. The shufflon is involved in the synthesis of PilV adhesins, which are responsible for recipient recognition in the conjugation process [53]. The insertion of IS*Ecp1*-*bla*$_{CTX-M-1}$ associated with the shuffling of segments can affect *PilV* and consequently modulate the recognition of recipient cells during IncI1-ST3-*bla*$_{CTX-M-1}$ conjugation. Resistance gene *bla*$_{CTX-M-1}$ can, therefore, be involved in both antimicrobial resistance and plasmid spread, two synergic functions that may explain the ecological success of *bla*$_{CTX-M-1}$ IncI1-ST3 plasmids.

5. Conclusions

Although additional animal and environmental sources of CTX-M-1-producing *E. coli* should be investigated, the results showed there was broad dissemination of IncI1-ST3-*bla*$_{CTX-M-1}$ plasmids. Their bacterial recipients differ by habitats, with a few of them playing the role of disseminating shuttles. The sequence of IncI1-ST3-*bla*$_{CTX-M-1}$ plasmids is highly conserved except in the shufflon zone. Their broad ecological success does not seem to be linked to their ability to transfer a broad spectrum of bacterial lineages, a feature associated with the diversity of their shuffling conjugation region.

Supplementary Materials: The following are available online at https://www.mdpi.com/article/10.3390/microorganisms9071471/s1, Figure S1: Frequency (a) and correlation index (b) of antimicrobial resistance genes in non-redundant *E. coli* harbouring *bla*$_{CTX-M-1}$ and IncI1-ST3 plasmids, Figure S2: Multiple corresponding analysis performed from the synteny of shuffling region of *bla*$_{CTX-M-1}$ IncI1-ST3 plasmids, Figure S3: Heatmap showing the presence (red) and the absence (blue) of synteny blocks in the shuffling region of plasmids IncI1-ST3-*bla*$_{CTX-M-1}$, Figure S4: Hierarchical classification of plasmids IncI1-ST3-*bla*$_{CTX-M-1}$ based on the synteny of the shufflon region, Table S1: Metadata associated with the *Escherichia coli* isolates sequenced during this study, Table S2: Dataset of *Escherichia coli* whole genome sequences (WGSs) containing replicon IncI1-ST3 encoding *bla*$_{CTX-M-1}$, Table S3: Circularised *bla*$_{CTX-M-1}$-encoding plasmids IncI1-ST3 included in this study.

Author Contributions: Conceptualisation, R.B. (Racha Beyrouthy) and R.B. (Richard Bonnet); methodology, R.B. (Racha Beyrouthy), and R.B. (Richard Bonnet); formal analysis, R.B., C.S., F.R., G.I. and P.P.; investigation, R.B. (Racha Beyrouthy), and R.B. (Richard Bonnet); resources, F.R., C.S., F.R., G.I. and P.P.; data curation, R.B. (Racha Beyrouthy), F.R. and R.B. (Richard Bonnet); writing—original draft preparation, R.B. (Racha Beyrouthy) and R.B. (Richard Bonnet); writing—review and editing, R.B. (Racha Beyrouthy) F.R., G.I., and R.B. (Richard Bonnet); supervision, R.B. (Racha Beyrouthy) and R.B. (Richard Bonnet); project administration, R.B. (Richard Bonnet); funding acquisition, R.B. (Richard Bonnet). All authors have read and agreed to the published version of the manuscript.

Funding: This study was funded by the Ministère de la Recherche et de la Technologie, Inserm (UMR 1071), INRAe (USC-2018), the French government's IDEX-ISITE initiative 16-IDEX-0001 (CAP 20-25) and by the JPIAMR program TransComp-ESC-R of the European Commission. We also thanks the "Espectrometria de massa e sequenciação aplicadas à microbiologia clínica moderna: pesquisa e identificação de biomarcadores em espécies bacterianas multiresistentes" (Programa de Acções Universitárias Integradas Luso-Francesas, Ação n.°: TC-14/2017) and by the Associate Laboratory for Green Chemistry-LAQV which is financed by national funds from FCT/MCTES (UID/QUI/50006/2019).

Institutional Review Board Statement: Not applicable.

Informed Consent Statement: Not applicable.

Data Availability Statement: The accession numbers of genomic data are reported in Supplementary Tables S2 and S3.

Acknowledgments: We thank Alexis Pontvianne and Lucie Pourpuech for their technical assistance.

Conflicts of Interest: The authors declare no conflict of interest.

References

1. Roca, I.; Akova, M.; Baquero, F.; Carlet, J.; Cavaleri, M.; Coenen, S.; Cohen, J.; Findlay, D.; Gyssens, I.; Heure, O.E.; et al. The global threat of antimicrobial resistance: Science for intervention. *New Microbes New Infect.* **2015**, *6*, 22–29. [CrossRef]
2. WHO. *WHO List of Critically Important Antimicrobials for Human Medicine (WHO CIA List)*; 5th Revision; World Health Organization: Geneva, Switzerland, 2017.
3. Frost, L.; Leplae, R.; Summers, A.; Toussaint, A. Mobile genetic elements: The agents of open source evolution. *Nat. Rev. Genet.* **2005**, *3*, 722–732. [CrossRef]
4. Queenan, A.M.; Bush, K. Carbapenemases: The versatile β-lactamases. *Clin. Microbiol. Rev.* **2007**, *20*, 440–458. [CrossRef] [PubMed]
5. Philippon, A.; Arlet, G.; Jacoby, G.A. Plasmid-determined AmpC-type β-lactamases. *Antimicrob. Agents Chemother.* **2002**, *46*, 1–11. [CrossRef] [PubMed]
6. Bonnet, R. Growing group of extended-spectrum β-lactamases: The CTX-M enzymes. *Antimicrob. Agents Chemother.* **2004**, *48*, 1–14. [CrossRef] [PubMed]
7. Paterson, D.L.; Bonomo, R.A. Extended spectrum beta lactamases: A critical update. *Clin. Microbiol. Rev.* **2005**, *18*, 657–686. [CrossRef]
8. Pitout, J.D.; Laupland, K.B. Extended-spectrum β-lactamase-producing Enterobacteriaceae: An emerging public-health concern. *Lancet Infect. Dis.* **2008**, *8*, 159–166. [CrossRef]
9. Bonomo, R.A.; Burd, E.M.; Conly, J.; Limbago, B.M.; Poirel, L.; Segre, J.A.; Westblade, L.F. Carbapenemase-producing organisms: A global scourge. *Clin. Infect. Dis.* **2018**, *66*, 1290–1297. [CrossRef]
10. David, S.; Reuter, S.; Harris, S.R.; Glasner, C.; Feltwell, T.; Argimon, S.; Abudahab, K.; Goater, R.; Giani, T.; Errico, G.; et al. Europe PMC funders group europe PMC funders author manuscripts Europe PMC funders author manuscripts epidemic of carbapenem-resistant Klebsiella pneumoniae in Europe is driven by nosocomial spread. *Nature* **2020**, *4*, 1919–1929.
11. Haenni, M.; Beyrouthy, R.; Lupo, A.; Châtre, P.; Madec, J.Y.; Bonnet, R. Epidemic spread of Escherichia coli ST744 isolates carrying mcr-3 and blaCTX-M-55 in cattle in France. *J. Antimicrob. Chemother.* **2018**, *73*, 533–536. [CrossRef]
12. Robin, F.; Beyrouthy, R.; Bonacorsi, S.; Aissa, N.; Bret, L.; Brieu, N.; Cattoir, V.; Chapuis, A.; Chardon, H.; Degand, N.; et al. Inventory of extended-spectrum-β-lactamase-producing enterobacteriaceae in France as assessed by a multicenter study. *Antimicrob. Agents Chemother.* **2017**, *61*, e01911-16. [CrossRef] [PubMed]
13. Wellington, E.M.; Boxall, A.B.; Cross, P.; Feil, E.J.; Gaze, W.H.; Hawkey, P.M.; Johnson-Rollings, A.S.; Jones, D.L.; Lee, N.M.; Otten, W.; et al. The role of the natural environment in the emergence of antibiotic resistance in Gram-negative bacteria. *Lancet Infect. Dis.* **2013**, *13*, 155–165. [CrossRef]
14. Pietsch, M.; Eller, C.; Wendt, C.; Holfelder, M.; Falgenhauer, L.; Fruth, A.; Grössl, T.; Leistner, R.; Valenza, G.; Werner, G.; et al. Molecular characterisation of extended-spectrum β-lactamase (ESBL)-producing Escherichia coli isolates from hospital and ambulatory patients in Germany. *Vet. Microbiol.* **2017**, *200*, 130–137. [CrossRef]
15. Liu, X.; Thungrat, K.; Boothe, D.M. Occurrence of oxa-48 carbapenemase and other β-lactamase genes in esbl-producing multidrug resistant: Escherichia coli from dogs and cats in the united states, 2009–2013. *Front. Microbiol.* **2016**, *7*, 1057. [CrossRef]
16. Götz, A.; Pukall, R.; Smit, E.; Tietze, E.; Prager, R.; Tschäpe, H.; van Elsas, J.D.; Smalla, K. Detection and characterization of broad-host-range plasmids in environmental bacteria by PCR. *Appl. Environ. Microbiol.* **1996**, *62*, 2621–2628. [CrossRef] [PubMed]
17. Pukall, R.; Tschäpe, H.; Smalla, K. Monitoring the spread of broad host and narrow host range plasmids in soil microcosms. *FEMS Microbiol. Ecol.* **1996**, *20*, 53–66. [CrossRef]
18. Dolejska, M.; Papagiannitsis, C.C. Plasmid-mediated resistance is going wild. *Plasmid* **2018**, *99*, 99–111. [CrossRef]
19. Carattoli, A.; Villa, L.; Fortini, D.; García-Fernández, A. Contemporary IncI1 plasmids involved in the transmission and spread of antimicrobial resistance in Enterobacteriaceae. *Plasmid* **2018**, 102392. [CrossRef]
20. Radhouani, H.; Pinto, L.; Coelho, C.; Gonçalves, A.; Sargo, R.; Torres, C.; Igrejas, G.; Poeta, P. Detection of Escherichia coli harbouring extended-spectrum β-lactamases of the CTX-M classes in faecal samples of common buzzards (*Buteo buteo*). *J. Antimicrob. Chemother.* **2010**, *65*, 171–173. [CrossRef]
21. Madec, J.Y.; Haenni, M.; Métayer, V.; Saras, E.; Nicolas-Chanoine, M.H. High prevalence of the animal-associated blaCTX-M-1 IncI1/ST3 plasmid in human Escherichia coli isolates. *Antimicrob. Agents Chemother.* **2015**, *59*, 5860–5861. [CrossRef]
22. Jakobsen, L.; Bortolaia, V.; Bielak, E.; Moodley, A.; Olsen, S.S.; Hansen, D.S.; Frimodt-Møller, N.; Guardabassi, L.; Hasman, H. Limited similarity between plasmids encoding CTX-M-1 β-lactamase in Escherichia coli from humans, pigs, cattle, organic poultry layers and horses in Denmark. *J. Glob. Antimicrob. Resist.* **2015**, *3*, 132–136. [CrossRef]
23. Carattoli, A. Resistance plasmid families in enterobacteriaceae. *Antimicrob. Agents Chemother.* **2009**, *53*, 2227–2238. [CrossRef]

24. Literak, I.; Dolejska, M.; Janoszowska, D.; Hrusakova, J.; Meissner, W.; Rzyska, H.; Bzoma, S.; Cizek, A. Antibiotic-resistant Escherichia coli bacteria, including strains with genes encoding the extended-spectrum beta-lactamase and QnrS, in waterbirds on the baltic sea coast of Poland. *Appl. Environ. Microbiol.* **2010**, *76*, 8126–8134. [CrossRef]
25. Veldman, K.; Van Tulden, P.; Kant, A.; Testerink, J.; Mevius, D. Characteristics of cefotaxime-resistant escherichia coli from wild birds in The Netherlands. *Appl. Environ. Microbiol.* **2013**, *79*, 7556–7561. [CrossRef]
26. Praszkier, J.; Pittard, A.J. Control of replication in I-complex plasmids. *Plasmid* **2005**, *53*, 97–112. [CrossRef] [PubMed]
27. Takahashi, H.; Shao, M.; Furuya, N.; Komano, T. The genome sequence of the incompatibility group Iγ plasmid R621a: Evolution of IncI plasmids. *Plasmid* **2011**, *66*, 112–121. [CrossRef] [PubMed]
28. Johnson, T.J.; Shepard, S.M.; Rivet, B.; Danzeisen, J.L.; Carattoli, A. Comparative genomics and phylogeny of the IncI1 plasmids: A common plasmid type among porcine enterotoxigenic Escherichia coli. *Plasmid* **2011**, *66*, 144–151. [CrossRef] [PubMed]
29. Hernando-Amado, S.; Coque, T.M.; Baquero, F.; Martínez, J.L. Defining and combating antibiotic resistance from One Health and Global Health perspectives. *Nat. Microbiol.* **2019**, *4*, 1432–1442. [CrossRef]
30. Huijbers, P.M.C.; Graat, E.A.M.; Haenen, A.P.J.; van Santen, M.G.; van Essen-Zandbergen, A.; Mevius, D.J.; Van Duijkeren, E.; Van Hoek, A.H.A.M. Extended-spectrum and AmpC β-lactamase-producing Escherichia coli in broilers and people living and/or working on broiler farms: Prevalence, risk factors and molecular characteristics. *J. Antimicrob. Chemother.* **2014**, *69*, 2669–2675. [CrossRef]
31. Ramos, S.; Silva, N.; Dias, D.; Sousa, M.; Capelo-Martínez, J.L.; Brito, F.; Caniça, M.; Igrejas, G.; Poeta, P. Clonal Diversity of ESBL-Producing Escherichia coli in Pigs at Slaughter Level in Portugal. *Foodborne Pathog. Dis.* **2013**, *10*, 74–79. [CrossRef]
32. Poeta, P.; Radhouani, H.; Pinto, L.; Martinho, A.; Rego, V.; Rodrigues, R.; Gonçalves, A.; Rodrigues, J.; Estepa, V.; Torres, C.; et al. Wild boars as reservoirs of extended-spectrum beta-lactamase (ESBL) producing Escherichia coli of different phylogenetic groups. *J. Basic Microbiol.* **2009**, *49*, 584–588. [CrossRef] [PubMed]
33. Poeta, P.; Radhouani, H.; Igrejas, G.; Gonçalves, A.; Carvalho, C.; Rodrigues, J.; Vinue, L.; Somalo, S.; Torres, C. Seagulls of the berlengas natural reserve of portugal as carriers of fecal escherichia coli harboring CTX-M and TEM extended-spectrum beta-lactamases. *Appl. Environ. Microbiol.* **2008**, *74*, 7439–7441. [CrossRef] [PubMed]
34. Pinto, L.; Radhouani, H.; Coelho, C.; Da Costa, P.M.; Simões, R.; Brandão, R.M.L.; Torres, C.; Igrejas, G.; Poeta, P. Genetic detection of extended-spectrum β-lactamase-containing Escherichia coli isolates from birds of prey from Serra da Estrela natural reserve in Portugal. *Appl. Environ. Microbiol.* **2010**, *76*, 4118–4120. [CrossRef] [PubMed]
35. Gonçalves, A.; Igrejas, G.; Radhouani, H.; Estepa, V.; Pacheco, R.; Monteiro, R.; Brito, F.; Guerra, A.; Petrucci-Fonseca, F.; Torres, C.; et al. Iberian wolf as a reservoir of extended-spectrum β-lactamase-producing escherichia coli of the TEM, SHV, and CTX-M groups. *Microb. Drug Resist.* **2012**, *18*, 215–219. [CrossRef] [PubMed]
36. Gonçalves, A.; Igrejas, G.; Radhouani, H.; Estepa, V.; Alcaide, E.; Zorrilla, I.; Serra, R.; Torres, C.; Poeta, P. Detection of extended-spectrum beta-lactamase-producing Escherichia coli isolates in faecal samples of Iberian lynx. *Lett. Appl. Microbiol.* **2011**, *54*, 73–77. [CrossRef]
37. Garcês, A.; Correia, S.; Amorim, F.; Pereira, J.; Igrejas, G.; Poeta, P. First report on extended-spectrum beta-lactamase (ESBL) producing Escherichia coli from European free-tailed bats (Tadarida teniotis) in Portugal: A one-health approach of a hidden contamination problem. *J. Hazard. Mater.* **2019**, *370*, 219–224. [CrossRef] [PubMed]
38. Chen, S.; Zhou, Y.; Chen, Y.; Gu, J. fastp: An ultra-fast all-in-one FASTQ preprocessor. *Bioinformatics* **2018**, *34*, i884–i890. [CrossRef]
39. Nurk, S.; Bankevich, A.; Antipov, D.; Gurevich, A.; Korobeynikov, A.; Lapidus, A.; Prjibelski, A.D.; Pyshkin, A.; Sirotkin, A.; Sirotkin, Y.; et al. Assembling single-cell genomes and mini-metagenomes from chimeric MDA products. *J. Comput. Biol.* **2013**, *20*, 714–737. [CrossRef] [PubMed]
40. Beghain, J.; Bridier-Nahmias, A.; Le Nagard, H.; Denamur, E.; Clermont, O. ClermonTyping: An easy-to-use and accurate in silico method for Escherichia genus strain phylotyping. *Microb. Genom.* **2018**, *4*, e000192. [CrossRef]
41. Wirth, T.; Falush, D.; Lan, R.; Colles, F.; Mensa, P.; Wieler, L.H.; Karch, H.; Reeves, P.R.; Maiden, M.C.J.; Ochman, H.; et al. Sex and virulence in Escherichia coli: An evolutionary perspective. *Mol. Microbiol.* **2006**, *60*, 1136–1151. [CrossRef]
42. Phan, M.D.; Peters, K.M.; Sarkar, S.; Lukowski, S.W.; Allsopp, L.P.; Moriel, D.G.; Achard, M.E.S.; Totsika, M.; Marshall, V.M.; Upton, M.; et al. The serum resistome of a globally disseminated multidrug resistant uropathogenic escherichia coli clone. *PLoS Genet.* **2013**, *9*, e1003834. [CrossRef] [PubMed]
43. Ben Zakour, N.L.; Alsheikh-Hussain, A.S.; Ashcroft, M.M.; Khanh Nhu, N.T.; Roberts, L.W.; Stanton-Cook, M.; Schembri, M.A.; Beatsona, S.A. Sequential acquisition of virulence and fluoroquinolone resistance has shaped the evolution of Escherichia coli ST131. *mBio* **2016**, *7*, e00347-16. [CrossRef] [PubMed]
44. Croucher, N.; Page, A.; Connor, T.; Delaney, A.J.; Keane, J.A.; Bentley, S.D.; Parkhill, J.; Harris, S.R. Rapid phylogenetic analysis of large samples of recombinant bacterial whole genome sequences using Gubbins. *Nucleic Acids Res.* **2015**, *43*, e15. [CrossRef] [PubMed]
45. Stamatakis, A. RAxML version 8: A tool for phylogenetic analysis and post-analysis of large phylogenies. *Bioinformatics* **2014**, *30*, 1312–1313. [CrossRef]
46. Jia, B.; Raphenya, A.R.; Alcock, B.; Waglechner, N.; Guo, P.; Tsang, K.K.; Lago, B.A.; Dave, B.M.; Pereira, S.; Sharma, A.N.; et al. CARD 2017: Expansion and model-centric curation of the comprehensive antibiotic resistance database. *Nucleic Acids Res.* **2017**, *45*, D566–D573. [CrossRef]

47. Zankari, E.; Hasman, H.; Cosentino, S.; Vestergaard, M.; Rasmussen, S.; Lund, O.; Aarestrup, F.; Larsen, M.V. Identification of acquired antimicrobial resistance genes. *J. Antimicrob. Chemother.* **2012**, *67*, 2640–2644. [CrossRef]
48. Beyrouthy, R.; Barets, M.; Marion, E.; Dananché, C.; Dauwalder, O.; Robin, F.; Gauthier, L.; Jousset, A.; Dortet, L.; Guérin, F.; et al. Novel enterobacter lineage as leading cause of nosocomial outbreak involving carbapenemase-producing strains. *Emerg. Infect. Dis.* **2018**, *24*, 1505–1515. [CrossRef]
49. Minkin, I.; Patel, A.; Kolmogorov, M.; Vyahhi, N.; Pham, S. Sibelia: A Scalable and Comprehensive Synteny Block Generation Tool for Closely Related Microbial Genomes. In *International Workshop on Algorithms in Bioinformatics*; Springer: Berlin/Heidelberg, Germany, 2013; Volume 8126, pp. 215–229.
50. Gyohda, A.; Furuya, N.; Kogure, N.; Komano, T. Sequence-specific and Non-specific binding of the rci protein to the asymmetric recombination sites of the R64 shufflon. *J. Mol. Biol.* **2002**, *318*, 975–983. [CrossRef]
51. Poirel, L.; Decousser, J.W.; Nordmann, P. Insertion sequence ISEcp1B is involved in expression and mobilization of a blaCTX-M β-lactamase gene. *Antimicrob. Agents Chemother.* **2003**, *47*, 2938–2945. [CrossRef]
52. Poirel, L.; Lartigue, M.-F.; Decousser, J.-W.; Nordmann, P. IS Ecp1B -Mediated Transposition of bla CTX-M in Escherichia coli. *Antimicrob. Agents Chemother.* **2005**, *49*, 447–450. [CrossRef] [PubMed]
53. Ishiwa, A.; Komano, T. Thin pilus Pilv adhesins of plasmid R64 recognize specific structures of the lipopolysaccharide molecules of recipient cells. *J. Bacteriol.* **2003**, *185*, 5192–5199. [CrossRef]
54. Liebana, E.; Carattoli, A.; Coque, T.M.; Hasman, H.; Magiorakos, A.P.; Mevius, D.; Peixe, L.; Poirel, L.; Schuepbach-Regula, G.; Torneke, K.; et al. Public health risks of enterobacterial isolates producing extended-spectrum β-lactamases or AmpC β-lactamases in food and food-producing animals: An EU perspective of epidemiology, analytical methods, risk factors, and control options. *Clin. Infect. Dis.* **2013**, *56*, 1030–1037. [CrossRef]
55. Jouini, A.; Ben Slama, K.; Klibi, N.; Ben Sallem, R.; Estepa, V.; Vinue, L.; Sáenz, Y.; Ruiz-Larrea, F.; Boudabous, A.; Torres, C. Lineages and Virulence Gene Content among Extended-Spectrum β-Lactamase–Producing Escherichia coli Strains of Food Origin in Tunisia. *J. Food Prot.* **2013**, *76*, 323–327. [CrossRef] [PubMed]
56. Day, M.J.; Hopkins, K.L.; Wareham, D.W.; Toleman, M.; Elviss, N.; Randall, L.; Teale, C.; Cleary, P.; Wiuff, C.; Doumith, M.; et al. Extended-spectrum β-lactamase-producing Escherichia coli in human-derived and foodchain-derived samples from England, Wales, and Scotland: An epidemiological surveillance and typing study. *Lancet Infect. Dis.* **2019**, *19*, 1325–1335. [CrossRef]
57. Irrgang, A.; Hammerl, J.A.; Falgenhauer, L.; Guiral, E.; Schmoger, S.; Imirzalioglu, C.; Fischer, J.; Guerra, B.; Chakraborty, T.; Käsbohrer, A. Diversity of CTX-M-1-producing E. coli from German food samples and genetic diversity of the blaCTX-M-1 region on IncI1 ST3 plasmids. *Vet. Microbiol.* **2018**, *221*, 98–104. [CrossRef] [PubMed]
58. Rodríguez-Beltrán, J.; DelaFuente, J.; León-Sampedro, R.; MacLean, R.C.; Millán, Á.S. Beyond horizontal gene transfer: The role of plasmids in bacterial evolution. *Nat. Rev. Genet.* **2021**, *19*, 347–359. [CrossRef] [PubMed]
59. Giles, W.P.; Benson, A.K.; Olson, M.E.; Hutkins, R.W.; Whichard, J.M.; Winokur, P.; Fey, P.D. DNA sequence analysis of regions surrounding blaCMY-2 from multiple salmonella plasmid backbones. *Antimicrob. Agents Chemother.* **2004**, *48*, 2845–2852. [CrossRef] [PubMed]
60. Sekizuka, T.; Kawanishi, M.; Ohnishi, M.; Shima, A.; Kato, K.; Yamashita, A.; Matsui, M.; Suzuki, S.; Kuroda, M. Elucidation of quantitative structural diversity of remarkable rearrangement regions, shufflons, in IncI2 plasmids. *Sci. Rep.* **2017**, *7*, 1–10. [CrossRef] [PubMed]
61. Sabença, C.; Igrejas, G.; Poeta, P.; Robin, F.; Bonnet, R.; Beyrouthy, R. Multidrug Resistance Dissemination in *Escherichia coli* isolated from wild animals: Bacterial clones and plasmid complicity. *Microbiol. Res.* **2021**, *12*, 9. [CrossRef]

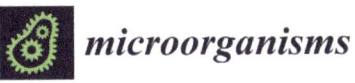

Article

Antibiotic Resistant and Biofilm-Associated *Escherichia coli* Isolates from Diarrheic and Healthy Dogs

Lívia Karahutová [1], René Mandelík [2] and Dobroslava Bujňáková [1,*]

1. Institute of Animal Physiology, Centre of Biosciences of the Slovak Academy of Sciences, Šoltésovej 4-6, 040 01 Košice, Slovakia; karahutova@saske.sk
2. Department of Epizootiology, Parasitology and Protection of One Health, University of Veterinary Medicine and Pharmacy in Košice, Komenského 73, 040 01 Košice, Slovakia; rene.mandelik@uvlf.sk
* Correspondence: dbujnak@saske.sk; Tel.: +421-55-727-62-76

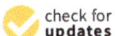

Citation: Karahutová, L.; Mandelík, R.; Bujňáková, D. Antibiotic Resistant and Biofilm-Associated *Escherichia coli* Isolates from Diarrheic and Healthy Dogs. *Microorganisms* 2021, 9, 1334. https://doi.org/10.3390/microorganisms9061334

Academic Editor: Charles M. Dozois

Received: 31 May 2021
Accepted: 16 June 2021
Published: 19 June 2021

Publisher's Note: MDPI stays neutral with regard to jurisdictional claims in published maps and institutional affiliations.

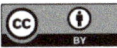

Copyright: © 2021 by the authors. Licensee MDPI, Basel, Switzerland. This article is an open access article distributed under the terms and conditions of the Creative Commons Attribution (CC BY) license (https://creativecommons.org/licenses/by/4.0/).

Abstract: Bacteria isolated from companion animals are attracting concerns in a view of public health including antimicrobial resistance and biofilm development, both contributing to difficult-to-treat infections. The purpose of this study was to evaluate the minimum inhibitory concentrations (MIC) of 18 antibiotics in *Escherichia coli* isolated from two groups of dogs (healthy and diarrheic). Isolates were classified into phylogroups, examined for the presence of resistance genes and biofilm-formation capacity. In healthy dogs, phylogenetic analysis showed that 47.37% and 34.22% of *E. coli* isolates belonged to commensal groups (A; B1) in contrast to diarrheic dogs; 42.2% of isolates were identified as the B2 phylogroup, and these *E. coli* bacteria formed a stronger biofilm. The results of healthy dogs showed higher MIC levels for tetracycline (32 mg/L), ampicillin (64 mg/L), ciprofloxacin (8 mg/L) and trimethoprim-sulphonamide (8 mg/L) compared to clinical breakpoints. The most detected gene encoding plasmid-mediated resistance to quinolones in the healthy group was *qnr*B, and in dogs with diarrhea, *qnr*S. The resistance genes were more frequently detected in healthy dogs. The presence of the integron *int1* and the transposon *tn3* increases the possibility of transfer of many different cassette-associated antibiotic-resistance genes. These results suggest that dogs could be a potential reservoir of resistance genes.

Keywords: *E. coli*; dogs; antimicrobial resistance; biofilm; phylogenetic groups

1. Introduction

Escherichia coli (*E. coli*) is a highly versatile bacterium that ranges from harmless gut commensal to intra- or extra- intestinal pathogens [1]. Commensal *E. coli* colonizes in the gastrointestinal tract within a few hours after birth. Although these strains are part of the normal microbiota of humans and animals, several clinical reports have implicated *E. coli* as the etiological agent of diarrhea in humans and their companion animals [2,3]. Previously, the most extensive investigations of *E. coli* infection have been described in cattle, sheep and pigs. However, recently, the dogs and cats that live in close proximity to humans have become a focus of disease transmission studies. Because the contact between humans and pets has increased, the possibility of pathogenic microorganism transmission between these organisms is very high. The fecal shedding of *E. coli* by companion animals represents an important source of the zoonotic transmission of pathogenic agents [2].

The prevalence of drug-resistant bacteria, caused among other things by an excessive use of antibiotics, is an increasing problem due to the possible transmission of resistant bacteria or their resistance genes between animals and humans via direct or indirect contact, such as through food/feed and the environment. Drug-resistant commensal *E. coli* isolates may constitute a significant reservoir of antibiotic-resistance determinants, which can spread to those bacteria that are pathogenic for animals and/or humans. Another problem is biofilm development, since the biofilm matrix gives an additional resistance power to the bacteria which makes them not only tolerant to harsh conditions but also resistant to antibiotics. This leads to the emergence of bad-bugs infections, such as multi-drug resistant, extensively drug resistant and totally drug resistant types of bacteria [4].

For a long time, the focus of research was mostly on antimicrobial resistance (AMR) monitoring in food-producing animals [5]. Recently, dogs and cats have been described as potential vehicles for AMR; however, the data remained scarce. Therefore, it was found necessary to take a closer look at the situation existing in companion animals. Furthermore, approaching any issue from a One Health perspective necessitates looking at the interactions between people, domestic animals including pets, wildlife, plants and our environment [6].

Dogs and cats represent potential sources for the spread of AMR, due to the extensive use of broad-spectrum antimicrobial agents in these animals (even those critically important for human medicine, such as third generation cephalosporins and fluoroquinolones, colistin, tetracyclines and macrolides) and their close and intensive contact with humans [7]. Moreover, pet feces on the ground of urban areas represent a significant public-health problem [8].

So far, especially within the European Union's member states, the monitoring of the existing situation concerning AMR in indicator bacteria such as *E. coli* of companion animals has been done sporadically. To the best of our knowledge, phenotypic resistance profiles of 282 *E. coli* isolates were determined to be present in dogs and cats in three European countries (Belgium, Italy and the Netherlands), of which 19% were isolated after antibiotic treatment of the monitored animals. Furthermore, the situation in Sweden [9] regards antibiotic resistance in the bacteria from humans and animals (including dogs), and a 331 indicator *E. coli* was mapped in the years 2006 and 2012. A similar situation exists throughout the European Union (EU) including the Slovak Republic, where the data on indicator *E. coli* isolates are only related to poultry and the meat derived thereof. A different situation is presented in the monitoring of AMR in clinical bacteria causing various infections [10]. However, studies of companion animals demonstrating the current situation of AMR concerning the indicator *E. coli* in the EU including the Slovak Republic are rather rare.

Therefore, the objectives of our study were to evaluate the phenotypic and genotypic AMR of commensal indicator and diarrheic *E. coli* isolated from Slovakian canine fecal samples using the standardized automated diagnostic system Bel-MIDITECH to classify their phylogenetic relatedness and to determine their biofilm-forming capacity as one of the factors contributing to increased resilience.

2. Materials and Methods

2.1. Canine Samples, Isolation and Identification of E. coli

The rectal swabs from 38 healthy non-antimicrobial treated dogs and 45 dogs with diarrhea, of varying breeds and from different households, were inoculated overnight at 37 °C in buffered peptone water (Oxoid, Basingstoke, UK). The samples from the diarrheal dogs were taken before an antibiotic treatment. The samples were then subcultured on MacConkey Agar (Oxoid, Basingstoke, UK) and UriSelect Agar (Bio-Rad Laboratories, Hercules, CA, USA) overnight at 37 °C. The colonies were isolated, identified and confirmed as *E. coli* using the MALDI–TOF MS (Matrix-Assisted Laser Desorption Ionization–Time of Flight, Mass Spectrometry) biotyper (Bruker Daltonics, Bremen, Germany) according to the methods described by Bessède et al. [11] and ENTEROtest24 (Erba Lachema Brno, Czech Republic) for the routine identification of important species of the Enterobacterales family within 24 h. One colony of *E. coli* was isolated from each sample.

2.2. Phylogenetic Groups

The form of the phylogenetic analysis was determined by using a new method, according to Clermont et al. [12]. The quadruplex polymerase chain reaction (PCR) was used to determine the phylogroup of each of the 83 isolates corresponding to the presence or absence of the genes *arp*A, *chu*A, *yja*A and *Tsp*E4.C2. All the isolates assigned to phylogroup

A were screened using a C-specific primer *trp*A (trpAgpC). Similarly, all the D phylogroup isolates were screened using an E-specific primer *arp*A (ArpAgpE). The oligonucleotide primers, annealing and references are listed in Table 1.

Table 1. Primers used for the PCR detection of resistance genes and phylogroups.

Gene	Primer Sequences (5′–3′)	Annealing (°C)	Size Product (bp)	Reference
int1	F:GGGTCAAGGATCTGGATTTCG R:ACATGCGTGTAAATCATCGTCG	62	483	[13]
tn3	F:CACGAATGAGGGCCGACAGGA R:ACCCACTCGTGCACCCAACTG	58	500	[14]
dfrA	F:GTGAAACTATCACTAATGG R:TTAACCCTTTTGCCAGATTT	55	474	[15]
dfrB	F:GATCGCCTGCGCAAGAAATC R:AAGCGCAGCCACAGGATAAAT	60	141	[15]
tetA	F:GGCCTCAATTTCCTGACG R:AAGCAGGATGTAGCCTGTGC	55	372	[16]
tetB	F:GAGACGCAATCGAATTCGG R:TTTAGTGGCTATTCTTCCTGCC	55	228	[16]
oqxA	F:GACAGCGTCGCACAGAATG R:GGAGACGAGGTTGGTATGGA	62	339	[17]
oqxB	F:CGAAGAAAGACCTCCCTACCC R:CGCCGCCAATGAGATACA	62	240	[17]
qepA	F:GCAGGTCCAGCAGCGGGTAG R:CTTCCTGCCCGAGTATCGTG	60	199	[18]
qnrS	F:ACGACATTCGTCAACTGCAA R:TAAATTGGCACCCTGTAGGC	53	417	[19]
qnrA	F:ATTTCTCACGCCAGGATTTG R:GATCGGCAAAGGTTAGGTCA	53	516	[19]
qnrB	F:GATCGTGAAAGCCAGAAAGG R:ACGATGCCTGGTAGTTGTCC	53	469	[19]
aac(6′)-Ib-cr	F:GATCTCATATCGTCGAGTGGTGG R:GAACCATGTACACGGCTGGAC	58	435	[19]
mcr-1	F:CGGTCAGTCCGTTTGTTC R:CTTGGTCGGTCTGTAGGG	58	309	[20]
mcr-2	F: TGTTGCTTGTGCCGATTGGA R:AGATGGTATTGTTGGTTGCTG	58	567	[21]
sul1	F:CGGCGTGGGCTACCTGAACG R:GCCGATCGCGTGAAGTTCCG	69	433	[22]
sul2	F:GCGCTCAAGGCAGATGGCATT R:GCGTTTGATACCGGCACCCGT	69	293	[22]
sul3	F: GAGCAAGATTTTTGGAATCG R:CATCTGCAGCTAACCTAGGGCTTTGA	51	990	[23]
arpA	F:AACGCTATTCGCCAGCTTGC R:TCTCCCCATACCGTACGCTA	59	400	[12]
chuA	F:ATGGTACCGGACGAACCAAC R:TGCCGCCAGTACCAAAGACA	59	288	[12]
yjaA	F:CAAACGTGAAGTGTCAGGAG R: AATGCGTTCCTCAACCTGTG	59	211	[12]
TspE4.C2	F: CACTATTCGTAAGGTCATCC R: AGTTTATCGCTGCGGGTCGC	59	152	[12]
arpAgpE	F:GATTCCATCTTGTCAAAATATGCC R:GAAAAGAAAAAGAATTCCCAAGAG	57	301	[24]
trpAgpC	F:AGTTTTATGCCCAGTGCGAG R:TCTGCGCCGGTCACGCCC	59	219	[24]
bla$_{TEM-1}$	F:ATGAGTATTCAACATTTCCG R:CCAATGCTTAATCAGTGAGG	55	858	[25]
bla$_{SHV}$	F:ATGCGTTATATTCGCCTGTG R:TTAGCGTTGCCAGTGCTCGATG	58	301	[26]
cit	F: TGGCCAGAACTGACAGGCAAA R: TTTCTCCTGAACGTGGCTGGC	64	462	[27]

Abbreviations: *int1* = integron; *tn3* = transposon; resistance to trimethoprim = *dfrA*, *dfrB*; resistance to tetracycline = *tetA*, *tetB*; quinolone resistance = *oqxA*, *oqxB*, aac(6′)-Ib-cr, *qepA*, *qnrS*, *qnrA*, *qnrB*; resistance to colistin = *mcr-1*, *mcr-2*; sulfonamide resistance = *sul1*, *sul2* and *sul3*; β-lactamase encoding *bla*$_{TEM-1}$, *bla*$_{SHV}$ and ampicillinase–cit. Phylogenetic grouping: *arpA*, *chuA*, *yjaA*, DNA fragment TspE4.C2 and requires additional testing for specific genes in the E (*arpAgpE*) and C (*trpAgpC*) groups.

2.3. Antimicrobial Sensitivity

The minimum inhibitory concentration (MIC) testing was performed according to Gattringer et al. [28] using the Slovakian automated diagnostic system Bel-MIDITECH (Bratislava, Slovakia) consisting of ampicillin (AMP), ampicillin + sulbactam (SAM), piperacillin + tazobactam (TZP), cefuroxime (CXM), cefotaxime (CTX), ceftazidime (CAZ), cefoperazone + sulbactam (SPZ), cefepime (FEP), ertapenem (ETP), meropenem (MEM), gentamicin (GEN), tobramycin (TOB), amikacin (AMI), tigecycline (TGC), ciprofloxacin (CIP), tetracycline (TET), colistin (COL) and trimethoprim + sulfonamide (COT). The results of the MIC values of each antibiotic were interpreted according to the clinical breakpoints (CBPs) described by The European Committee on Antimicrobial Susceptibility Testing (EUCAST) 2020 [29].

2.4. Detection of Resistance Genes

The strains were investigated for the presence of resistance genes using primers, as shown in Table 1, by means of multiplex and/or single PCR assays. The amplifications were carried out in a single tube with a volume of 25 µL, utilizing TaqI polymerase (Solis Biodyne, Estonia) with $10 \times$ Buffer B without Mg^{2+} (2–2.5 µL); deoxynucleotide triphosphates (dNTPs) mix (Promega, Madison, WI, USA; 2.5 µL); 25 mM $MgCl_2$ (1.5–2.5 µL); 10–20 pmol/µL primers (Lambda Life, Bratislava, Slovakia; 0.1–0.2 µL); 10–100 ng/µL DNA template (1–1.5 µL); and deionized sterile water. The PCR program consisted of an initial denaturation step at 95 °C for 4 min, followed by 32 cycles of DNA denaturation at 95 °C for 50 s, primer annealing at 50–69 °C (according to primers) for 50 s and primer extension at 72 °C for 1 min. After the last cycle, a final extension step at 72 °C for 7 min was added. The presence of genes for a resistance to trimethoprim–dihydrofolate reductase enzymes *dfr*A and *dfr*B; sulfonamide resistance–*sul1*, *sul2* and *sul3*; resistance to tetracycline—*tet*A and *tet*B; quinolone resistance–*oqx*A, *oqx*B; additional plasmid mediated quinolone resistance determinants–*aac* (6′)-*Ib-cr*; quinolone extrusion by *qep*A, *qnr*S, *qnr*A and *qnr*B; resistance to colistin encoded by *mcr-1* and *mcr-2*; β-lactamase encoding bla_{TEM-1}, bla_{SHV} and ampicillinase–*cit* were monitored. Moreover, we evaluated the presence of genes for integron *int1* and transposon *tn3*, because they are capable of capturing and expressing the genes contained in cassette-like structures that represent a substantial proportion of the resistance determinants in Gram-negative bacteria.

2.5. Detection of Biofilm Formation

The ability for biofilm formation was assessed in a quantitative assay using a microtiterplate test (Nunc, Roskilde, Denmark). Strains were grown on Brain Heart Infusion (BHI) agar, and colonies were re-suspended in a BHI broth (Oxoid, Basingstoke, UK) to reach the 0.5 suspension of McFarland's standard, and volumes of 200 µL of these cell suspensions were transferred to the wells of the microplate. For the negative control, we used an uninoculated BHI medium. After incubation (24 h at 37 °C), the adherent cells were washed three times using a saline solution and stained with a 0.1% crystal violet solution (Mikrochem, Pezinok, Slovakia). The adhering dye was dissolved with 30% acetic acid, and the optical density was measured at 570 nm in the Synergy HT Multi-Mode Microplate Reader (BioTek, Winooski, VT, USA). For classification, we used the average optical density (OD) value and cut-off value (ODc) (defined as three standard deviations (SD) above the mean OD of the negative control). The final OD value of a tested strain was expressed as the average OD value of the strain reduced by the ODc value. For the interpretation of the results, the strains were divided into the categories described by Stepanovic et al. [30]: OD $\leq$ ODc = non-biofilm producer; ODc < OD $\leq 2 \times$ ODc = weak biofilm; $2 \times$ ODc < OD $\leq \times$ ODc = moderate and $4 \times$ ODc < OD = strong biofilm producer.

3. Results and Discussion

3.1. Antimicrobial Sensitivity

A total of 38 *E. coli* isolates recovered from the fecal samples of healthy non-antimicrobial treated dogs and 45 *E. coli* isolates from dogs with diarrhea were investigated to phenotypic and genotypic antimicrobial resistance profiles.

In our study, the highest frequency of resistance in the healthy dogs was recorded for tetracycline ($n = 13$), ampicillin ($n = 12$), ciprofloxacin ($n = 6$), ampicillin + sulbactam ($n = 6$) and trimethoprim + sulphonamide ($n = 5$). This resistance phenotype is the most common, and this could indicate the mobile nature of the genes responsible for these resistance phenotypes [31]. Two of the isolates showed phenotypic colistin resistance.

The group of dogs with diarrhea showed a lower resistance profile for ampicillin ($n = 0$), ampicillin + sulbactam ($n = 2$) and trimethoprim + sulphonamide ($n = 4$). Only their resistance to ciprofloxacin ($n = 12$) and tetracycline ($n = 14$) was higher.

These findings are important for clinicians because β-lactam antibiotics are the most frequently used antimicrobials for gastrointestinal disease in dogs and cats [32]. Ampicillin-resistant *E. coli* could still be isolated from the dogs treated with antibiotics 21 days after treatment [33]. This emphasizes the fact that the intestinal tract acts as a reservoir for resistant bacteria long after the treatment has been stopped. Different studies suggest that high levels of resistance genes can still be found up to four years after antibiotic exposure [34,35]. This once more supports the importance of prudent antimicrobial usage in order to prevent the spread of antibiotic resistance.

3.2. Interpretative Reading of the Antibiogram and Detection of Resistance Genes

The most commonly used antimicrobials for companion animals in Europe (e.g., Poland [36], Italy [37], Finland [38], Sweden [39], Norway [40] and the UK [41]) are β-lactams (such as ampicillin, amoxicillin and amoxicillin-clavulanate). Fluoroquinolones, macrolides, tetracyclines, nitroimidazoles and trimethoprim/sulphonamides have been also reported to be routinely used in small animal practice, but on a much smaller scale than β-lactams.

Resistance to ampicillin (AMP) was found in 12 of the *E. coli* isolated from healthy animals. The value of MIC 90 (minimum inhibitory concentration required to inhibit the growth of 90% of microorganisms) for AMP in this group was 64 mg/L. Compared to the EUCAST clinical breakpoint (CBP) (AMP = 8 mg/L), the level of our MIC was very high. Next, a very important antibiotic for this group is ampicillin + sulbactam (SAM), because it has a good safety profile and provides coverage for a wide spectrum of bacterial pathogens. Six isolates from the healthy dogs were resistant to SAM, with a MIC 90 (16 mg/L) value slightly lower than for AMP (CBP for SAM = 8 mg/L), while only two such isolates were found in the dogs with diarrhea (MIC 90 = 8 mg/L). These results are comparable with other studies conducted in Europe [42,43], although a higher resistance is more often reported in southern European countries [10], which supports the importance of detecting the antibiotic profile for success treatment in companion animals. From the β-lactamase genes, we detected only simple bla_{TEM-1} in six isolates from the healthy dogs.

Some of the MIC levels found in this study were worrisome. The target MIC value for colistin (COL) is 4 mg/L, or exceptionally 2 mg/L. An interesting finding was the detection of phenotypic colistin-resistance in our two strains from healthy dogs, specifically with values of 4 mg/L and 8 mg/L and one isolate from the dogs with diarrhea (8 mg/L). For a further study of the mechanism of this type of resistance, it is recommended that a molecular method should be used for the detection of the *mcr-1* and *mcr-2* genes; however, in our case, this has not been confirmed. To the best of our knowledge, COL resistance in companion animals has only been described in China [44], Germany [45], Finland [46], Ecuador [47] and the Netherlands [43]. COL is currently the last choice in the treatment of human infections caused by carbapenem-resistant enterobacteria.

The presence of tetracycline (TET) resistance was detected in the *E. coli* of both healthy ($n = 13$) and sick dogs ($n = 14$) with MIC 90 (32 mg/L). Similarly, relatively high levels of TET resistance have been documented in other studies of dogs; for example, in Italy, Belgium and the Netherlands [43] as well as in Poland [36]. In the past, tetracycline has been used not only to treat urinary tract infections (UTIs), but various derivates of TET (such as chlortetracycline) have been used as a growth promotor [48], and the resistance probably reflects the long history of this application. These results indicate that the resistance to TET is still growing, and it should be used only if the susceptibility of the bacteria is confirmed by an in vitro study. Resistance to TET is conferred by one or more of the described *tet* genes, which encode one of three resistance and efflux mechanisms that appear to be more abundant among Gram-negative microorganisms [49]. All of our isolates were examined for the presence of *tet*A and/or *tet*B genes. The most common determinant in the healthy isolates was the *tet*A gene ($n = 19$), while *tet*B was detected in five isolates. These results are comparable with others described by Costa et al., Torkan et al. and Yousefi et al. [50–52]. On the other hand, the isolates from dogs with diarrhea showed a higher prevalence of the *tet*B gene ($n = 13$) versus *tet*A ($n = 5$).

Fluoroquinolone resistance is multifactorial, with both chromosomal and plasmid-mediated quinolone resistance (PMQR) mechanisms that are often contributing to the overall MIC [53]. The emergence of PMQR indicates that quinolone resistance can also be acquired through a horizontal gene transfer [54], and PMQR genes can create an environment in *E. coli* for the rapid selection of high levels of resistance [55]. The MIC 90 of ciprofloxacin (CIP) was MIC 90 = 8 mg/L in both groups (Figure 1) and was higher than CBP (0.5 mg/L). Among the 38 healthy *E. coli* isolates, 16 carried PMQR genes including the *qnr*B gene in 13 isolates, *qnr*S in two isolates and one isolate with *aac(6′)-Ib-cr*. The isolates from dogs with diarrhea were positive for *qnr*S ($n = 9$) and *aac(6′)-Ib-cr* ($n = 2$). As in other studies [56,57], genes encoding PMQR were also present in the ciprofloxacin-sensitive isolates, and this was not only related to the selective pressure of the fluoroquinolones used.

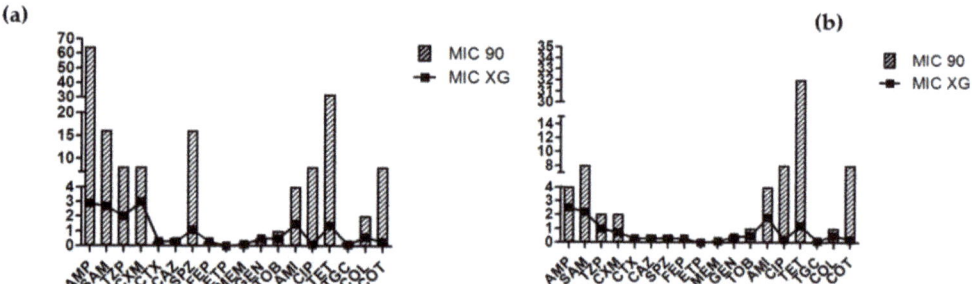

Figure 1. The values of MIC 90 and MIC XG (geometric mean MIC values of an antibiotic agent; mg/L) in *E. coli* of (**a**) healthy dogs and (**b**) dogs with diarrhea. Abbreviations: AMP = ampicillin; SAM = ampicillin + sulbactam; TZP = piperacillin + tazobactam; CXM = cefuroxime; CTX = cefotaxime; CAZ = ceftazidime; SPZ = cefoperazone + sulbactam; FEP = cefepime; ETP = ertapenem; MEM = meropenem; GEN = gentamicin; TOB = tobramycin; AMI = amikacin; CIP = ciprofloxacin; TET = tetracycline; TGC = tigecycline; COL = colistin and COT = trimethoprim + sulfonamide.

Resistance to trimethoprim-sulphonamide (COT) was detected in 11 *E. coli* strains from the healthy dogs and 5 isolates from the diarrheal dogs. In this study, the trimethoprim determinant *dfr*A was harbored by three isolates of the healthy dogs. This rate of COT resistance gene acquisition is high, and may be due to selection resulting from the frequent use of the sulfonamide/trimethoprim combination (due to its broad-spectrum activity) in small animal medicine [51]. This may also explain the presence of *sul1* ($n = 1$ in the healthy dogs) and *sul2* ($n = 9$ in the healthy dogs and $n = 5$ in the dogs with diarrhea) genes in our examined isolates. These results indicate a transmission of resistance genes to the normal microflora of healthy dogs.

Antimicrobial multidrug resistance (MDR) (resistance to at the least three different classes of antibiotics) was reported in 11 isolates of the healthy dogs and 2 isolates of the diarrheal dogs. The presence of integron 1 (*int1*; *n* = 12) and transposome (*tn3*; *n* = 12) in the healthy dogs indicates that the genetic mechanism for obtaining AMR genes is present not only in clinically-obtained isolates, but also in the isolates of a normal pet's microbiota. The *int1* gene often occurs in combination with trimethoprim resistance (*dfr*) and resistance to sulphonamide (*sul*), and it was detected in two isolates from the healthy dogs.

Data on pet animals is clearly needed for guiding the antimicrobial use policies in small animal veterinary practice, as well as for assessing the risk of the transmission of antimicrobial resistance to humans. Although our work evaluated antibiotic resistance without comparing our isolates to human ones, there are other existing studies that provide support for the occasional cross-host-species sharing of resistant strains, which highlights the importance of understanding the role of companion animals in the overall transmission patterns of multi-drug resistant *E. coli* with the potential for causing intestinal and/or extraintestinal infection [58,59].

3.3. Phylogenetic Analysis and Biofilm Formation

Focusing on the phylogenetic analysis (Figure 2), most of the strains from the healthy dog group were classified into commensal intestinal groups. In detail, 18 isolates were members of phylogroup A, and 13 were members of phylogroup B1. Pathogenic phylogroups occurred less frequently, but phylogroup B2 included three isolates; phylogroup E consisted of two isolates; one isolate fell into each of the phylogroup D and F groups.

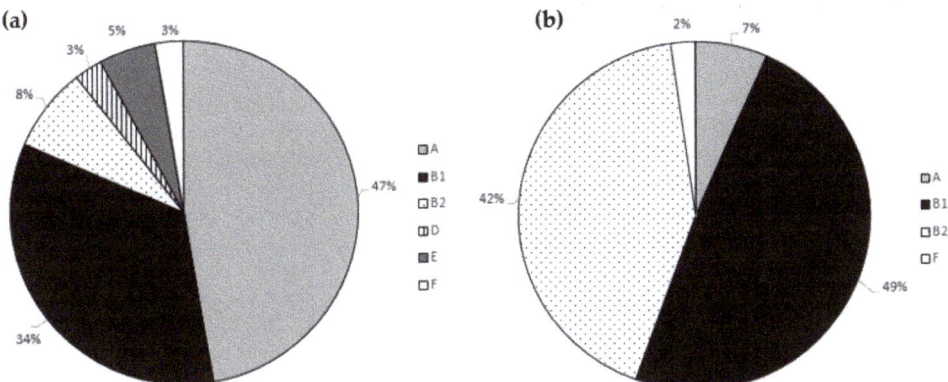

Figure 2. The *E. coli* phylogroup analysis in (**a**) healthy dogs and (**b**) dogs with diarrhea.

The many strains from the dogs with diarrhea were classified into B2 (19/45; 42.2%) and B1 (22/45; 48.90%) groups. Our comparative analysis between the phylogroups of the healthy and diarrheic dogs showed that the phylogroup B2 was visibly more common in the dogs with diarrhea.

In the healthy animals, the B1 group predominated, followed by the A, B2 and D groups [60]. These findings are important and show that the healthy dogs are colonized by commensal and pathogenic strains. The observation that the phylogenetic group B2 was usually related with the uropathogenic *E. coli* (UPEC) infection and the phylogenetic group D with the other extraintestinal pathogenic *E. coli* (ExPEC) has been previously reported [61,62]. Our results are comparable with those of Vega-Manriquez et al. [63], where the phylogroup analysis showed that a greater half (57%) of the *E. coli* isolates from the healthy dogs belonged to the commensal A and B1 groups, in contrast to the sick dogs, where the phylogroups D and B2 were dominant. In a study by Valat et al. [64], most of the pathogenic *E. coli* in dogs from digestive pathologies were also assigned to the B2 phylogroup (58.6%).

The ability of *E. coli* to form a biofilm is an important virulent property. Our strains were divided into four main groups on the basis of their biofilm-producing capacity (Figure 3).

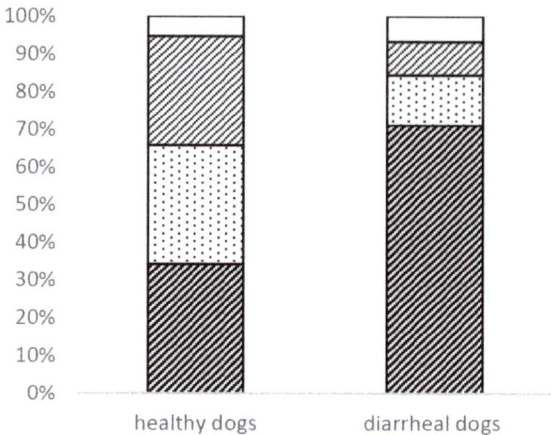

Figure 3. The ability of *E. coli* isolates to form biofilm.

In the healthy dogs, 13 strains (34.2%) were classified as strong biofilm producers, while the remaining 12 strains (31.6%) were regarded as moderate and 11 (29%) as weak biofilm producers. Only two of the strains did not form a biofilm. Most of the clinical isolates (70%, n = 32) had a stronger ability to form biofilms, followed by 13% moderate and 9% weak biofilm producers. In their study, Vijay et al. [65] examined the ability to form a biofilm in enteroaggregative *E. coli* (EAEC) from humans and animals with diarrhea. In that case, the EAEC isolates recovered from animals were low biofilm producers (65.3%), followed by moderate (26.5%) and high biofilm producers (8.1%). It has been reported [66,67] that biofilm formation may be an important contributory factor in persistent infection, either by allowing the bacteria to evade the local immune system and/or by preventing the transport of antibacterial factors, including antibiotics.

The analysis between the phylogenetic groups and the presence of phenotypic AMR (Table 2) shows that 17 *E. coli* of the healthy dogs belonging to the commensal phylogenetic groups—A, B1—were without AMR phenotypic profile along with all examined strains belong to the pathogenic groups B2, D, E and F. The remaining 14 *E. coli*—part of the commensal phylogroups—showed resistance to antibiotics. The most common phenotypic AMR profile in the healthy dogs were AMP–TET–COT (phylogroup A = 2 isolates; B1 = 2 isolates) and AMP–CIP–TET–COT (phylogroup A = 2 isolates; B1 = 2 isolates). Twenty-three *E. coli* of the sick dogs belonging to the commensal phylogenetic groups— A, B1—were without AMR phenotypic profile, and two isolates showed phenotypic resistance only to colistin. Predominant isolates of dogs with diarrhea showed the most common form of CIP—TET combination in the B2 phylogroup (n = 7). Our study compared the values of MIC 90 and MIC XG (geometric mean MIC values of an antibiotic agent; mg/L) in *E. coli* of healthy dogs and dogs with diarrhea and points only to a slight increase in these values in healthy animals versus dogs with diarrhea.

Table 2. The frequency of phenotypic antimicrobial resistance/sensitivity divided into phylogroups in healthy and sick dogs.

Phylogroups of Healthy Dogs	Phenotypic Antimicrobial Resistance Profile	Number of Isolates
A	Without AMR profile	$n = 8$
A	TET	$n = 2$
A	AMP, COT	$n = 1$
A	AMP, TET, COT	$n = 2$
A	AMP, SAM, TET	$n = 1$
A	AMP, CIP, TET, COT	$n = 2$
A	AMP, CIP, TET, COL, COT	$n = 2$
B1	Without AMR profile	$n = 9$
B1	AMP, TET, COT	$n = 2$
B1	AMP, CIP, TET, COT	$n = 2$
B2	Without AMR profile	$n = 3$
D	Without AMR profile	$n = 1$
E	Without AMR profile	$n = 2$
F	Without AMR profile	$n = 1$
Phylogroups of sick dogs	Phenotypic antimicrobial resistance profile	Number of isolates
A	Without AMR profile	$n = 3$
B1	Without AMR profile	$n = 20$
B1	COL	$n = 2$
B2	CIP	$n = 4$
B2	TET	$n = 3$
B2	CIP, TET	$n = 7$
B2	TET, COT	$n = 2$
B2	CIP, COT	$n = 1$
B2	SAM, TET, COT	$n = 2$
F	Without AMR profile	$n = 1$

Abbreviations: AMP = ampicillin; SAM = ampicillin + sulbactam; CIP = ciprofloxacin; TET = tetracycline; COL = colistin and COT = trimethoprim + sulfonamide.

4. Conclusions

This study reported on a comparison of *E. coli* isolates from healthy and diarrheic dogs. The observed results in the dogs with diarrhea showed differences in the phylogenetic representation, especially in terms of a high incidence of B2 isolates that were able to form a stronger biofilm compared to isolates from healthy dogs. The MIC 90 and MIC XG monitoring pointed out only a slight increase in these values in healthy animals. However, a high prevalence of genes encoding AMR and mobile elements in commensal *E. coli* can indicate that these strains can be a vehicle for the spread dissemination of AMR.

Author Contributions: Conceptualization, D.B., L.K.; methodology, L.K.; validation, D.B., L.K.; writing—original draft preparation, L.K., D.B., R.M.; writing—review and editing, D.B.; supervision, D.B.; resources of isolates, R.M.; project administration, D.B.; funding acquisition, D.B. All authors have read and agreed to the published version of the manuscript.

Funding: This research was funded by VEGA grant number 2/0010/21 and Cost Action CA18217 (European Network for Optimization of Veterinary Antimicrobial Treatment).

Conflicts of Interest: The authors declare no conflict of interest. The funders had no role in the design of the study; in the collection, analyses or interpretation of data; in the writing of the manuscript or in the decision to publish the results.

References

1. Kaper, J.B.; Nataro, J.P.; Mobley, H.L.T. Pathogenic *Escherichia coli*. *Nat. Rev. Microbiol.* **2004**, *2*, 123–140. [CrossRef]
2. Puño-Sarmiento, J.; Medeiros, L.; Chiconi, C.; Martins, F.; Pelayo, J.; Rocha, S.; Blanco, J.; Blanco, M.; Zanutto, M.; Kobayashi, R.; et al. Detection of Diarrheagenic *Escherichia coli* Strains Isolated from Dogs and Cats in Brazil. *Vet. Microbiol.* **2013**, *166*, 676–680. [CrossRef] [PubMed]
3. Majowicz, S.E.; Scallan, E.; Jones-Bitton, A.; Sargeant, J.M.; Stapleton, J.; Angulo, F.J.; Yeung, D.H.; Kirk, M.D. Global Incidence of Human Shiga Toxin–Producing *Escherichia coli* Infections and Deaths: A Systematic Review and Knowledge Synthesis. *Foodborne Pathog. Dis.* **2014**, *11*, 447–455. [CrossRef] [PubMed]
4. Sharma, D.; Misba, L.; Khan, A.U. Antibiotics versus Biofilm: An Emerging Battleground in Microbial Communities. *Antimicrob. Resist. Infect. Control* **2019**, *8*, 76. [CrossRef] [PubMed]
5. Ferreira, J.P.; Staerk, K. Antimicrobial Resistance and Antimicrobial Use Animal Monitoring Policies in Europe: Where Are We? *J. Public Health Policy* **2017**, *38*, 185–202. [CrossRef]
6. Collignon, P.; McEwen, S. One Health—Its Importance in Helping to Better Control Antimicrobial Resistance. *Trop. Med. Infect. Dis.* **2019**, *4*, 22. [CrossRef] [PubMed]
7. Guardabassi, L.; Schwarz, S.; Lloyd, D.H. Pet Animals as Reservoirs of Antimicrobial-Resistant BacteriaReview. *J. Antimicrob. Chemother.* **2004**, *54*, 321–332. [CrossRef] [PubMed]
8. Penakalapati, G.; Swarthout, J.; Delahoy, M.J.; McAliley, L.; Wodnik, B.; Levy, K.; Freeman, M.C. Exposure to Animal Feces and Human Health: A Systematic Review and Proposed Research Priorities. *Environ. Sci. Technol.* **2017**, *51*, 11537–11552. [CrossRef]
9. Swedres-Svarm 2019. Sales of Antibiotics and Occurrence of Resistance in Sweden. Solna/Uppsala ISSN1650-6332. Available online: www.sva.se/swedres-svarm/ (accessed on 19 March 2021).
10. The European Union Summary Report on Antimicrobial Resistance in Zoonotic and Indicator Bacteria from Humans, Animals and Food in 2014. *EFSA J.* **2016**, *14*. [CrossRef]
11. Bessède, E.; Angla-Gre, M.; Delagarde, Y.; Hieng, S.S.; Ménard, A.; Mégraud, F. Matrix-Assisted Laser-Desorption/Ionization Biotyper: Experience in the Routine of a University Hospital. *Clin. Microbiol. Infect.* **2011**, *17*, 533–538. [CrossRef] [PubMed]
12. Clermont, O.; Christenson, J.K.; Denamur, E.; Gordon, D.M. The Clermont *Escherichia coli* Phylo-Typing Method Revisited: Improvement of Specificity and Detection of New Phylo-Groups. *Environ. Microbiol. Rep.* **2013**, *5*, 58–65. [CrossRef]
13. Mazel, D.; Dychinco, B.; Webb, V.A.; Davies, J. Antibiotic Resistance in the ECOR Collection: Integrons and Identification of a Novel Aad Gene. *Antimicrob. Agents Chemother.* **2000**, *44*, 1568–1574. [CrossRef]
14. Weill, F.-X.; Demartin, M.; Fabre, L.; Grimont, P.A.D. Extended-Spectrum-β-Lactamase (TEM-52)-Producing Strains of *Salmonella enterica* of Various Serotypes Isolated in France. *J. Clin. Microbiol.* **2004**, *42*, 3359–3362. [CrossRef] [PubMed]
15. Navia, M.M.; Ruiz, J.; Sanchez-Cespedes, J.; Vila, J. Detection of Dihydrofolate Reductase Genes by PCR and RFLP. *Diagn. Microbiol. Infect. Dis.* **2003**, *46*, 295–298. [CrossRef]
16. Guillaume, G.; Verbrugge, D.; Chasseur-Libotte, M.-L.; Moens, W.; Collard, J.-M. PCR Typing of Tetracycline Resistance Determinants (Tet A–E) in *Salmonella enterica* Serotype Hadar and in the Microbial Community of Activated Sludges from Hospital and Urban Wastewater Treatment Facilities in Belgium. *FEMS Microbiol. Ecol.* **2000**, *32*, 77–85. [CrossRef] [PubMed]
17. Chen, X.; Zhang, W.; Pan, W.; Yin, J.; Pan, Z.; Gao, S.; Jiao, X. Prevalence of Qnr, Aac(6′)-Ib-Cr, QepA, and OqxAB in *Escherichia coli* Isolates from Humans, Animals, and the Environment. *Antimicrob. Agents Chemother.* **2012**, *56*, 3423–3427. [CrossRef]
18. Yamane, K.; Wachino, J.; Suzuki, S.; Arakawa, Y. Plasmid-Mediated QepA Gene among *Escherichia coli* Clinical Isolates from Japan. *Antimicrob. Agents Chemother.* **2008**, *52*, 1564–1566. [CrossRef]
19. Robicsek, A.; Strahilevitz, J.; Sahm, D.F.; Jacoby, G.A.; Hooper, D.C. Qnr Prevalence in Ceftazidime-Resistant Enterobacteriaceae Isolates from the United States. *Antimicrob. Agents Chemother.* **2006**, *50*, 2872–2874. [CrossRef]
20. Liu, Y.-Y.; Wang, Y.; Walsh, T.R.; Yi, L.-X.; Zhang, R.; Spencer, J.; Doi, Y.; Tian, G.; Dong, B.; Huang, X.; et al. Emergence of Plasmid-Mediated Colistin Resistance Mechanism MCR-1 in Animals and Human Beings in China: A Microbiological and Molecular Biological Study. *Lancet Infect. Dis.* **2016**, *16*, 161–168. [CrossRef]
21. Xavier, B.B.; Lammens, C.; Ruhal, R.; Kumar-Singh, S.; Butaye, P.; Goossens, H.; Malhotra-Kumar, S. Identification of a Novel Plasmid-Mediated Colistin-Resistance Gene, Mcr-2, in *Escherichia coli*, Belgium, June 2016. *Eurosurveillance* **2016**, *21*, 30280. [CrossRef]
22. Kerrn, M.B.; Klemmensen, T.; Frimodt-Møller, N.; Espersen, F. Susceptibility of Danish *Escherichia coli* Strains Isolated from Urinary Tract Infections and Bacteraemia, and Distribution of Sul Genes Conferring Sulphonamide Resistance. *J. Antimicrob. Chemother.* **2002**, *50*, 513–516. [CrossRef]
23. Guerra, B.; Junker, E.; Helmuth, R. Incidence of the Recently Described Sulfonamide Resistance Gene Sul3 among German *Salmonella enterica* Strains Isolated from Livestock and Food. *Antimicrob. Agents Chemother.* **2004**, *48*, 2712–2715. [CrossRef]
24. Lescat, M.; Clermont, O.; Woerther, P.L.; Glodt, J.; Dion, S.; Skurnik, D.; Djossou, F.; Dupont, C.; Perroz, G.; Picard, B.; et al. Commensal *Escherichia coli* Strains in Guiana Reveal a High Genetic Diversity with Host-Dependant Population Structure. *Environ. Microbiol. Rep.* **2013**, *5*, 49–57. [CrossRef] [PubMed]
25. Yates, C.; Brown, D.; Edwards, G.; Amyes, S. Detection of TEM-52 in *Salmonella enterica* Serovar Enteritidis Isolated in Scotland. *J. Antimicrob. Chemother.* **2004**, *53*, 407–408. [CrossRef] [PubMed]
26. Rodriguez-Villalobos, H.; Malaviolle, V.; Frankard, J.; de Mendonça, R.; Nonhoff, C.; Struelens, M.J. In Vitro Activity of Temocillin against Extended Spectrum Beta-Lactamase-Producing *Escherichia coli*. *J. Antimicrob. Chemother.* **2006**, *57*, 771–774. [CrossRef]

27. Pérez-Pérez, P.J.; Hanson, N.D. Detection of Plasmid-Mediated AmpC beta-Lactamase Genes in Clinical Isolates by Using Multiplex PCR. *J. Clin. Microbiol.* **2002**, *40*, 2153–2162. [CrossRef] [PubMed]
28. Gattringer, R.; Niks, M.; Ostertág, R.; Schwarz, K.; Medvedovic, H.; Graninger, W.; Georgopoulos, A. Evaluation of MIDITECH Automated Colorimetric MIC Reading for Antimicrobial Susceptibility Testing. *J. Antimicrob. Chemother.* **2002**, *49*, 651–659. [CrossRef]
29. The European Committee on Antimicrobial Susceptibility Testing. Breakpoint Tables for Interpretation of MICs and Zone Diameters, Version 10.0. 2020. Available online: https://www.eucast.org/fileadmin/src/media/PDFs/EUCAST_files/Resistance_mechanisms/EUCAST_detection_of_resistance_mechanisms_170711.pdf (accessed on 10 October 2020).
30. Stepanović, S.; Vuković, D.; Hola, V.; Bonaventura, G.D.; Djukić, S.; Ćirković, I.; Ruzicka, F. Quantification of Biofilm in Microtiter Plates: Overview of Testing Conditions and Practical Recommendations for Assessment of Biofilm Production by Staphylococci. *APMIS* **2007**, *115*, 891–899. [CrossRef]
31. Wedley, A.L.; Maddox, T.W.; Westgarth, C.; Coyne, K.P.; Pinchbeck, G.L.; Williams, N.J.; Dawson, S. Prevalence of Antimicrobial-Resistant *Escherichia coli* in Dogs in a Cross-Sectional, Community-Based Study. *Vet. Rec.* **2011**, *168*, 354. [CrossRef]
32. German, A.J.; Halladay, L.J.; Noble, P.-J.M. First-Choice Therapy for Dogs Presenting with Diarrhea in Clinical Practice. *Vet. Rec.* **2010**, *167*, 810–814. [CrossRef]
33. Werner, M.; Suchodolski, J.S.; Straubinger, R.K.; Wolf, G.; Steiner, J.M.; Lidbury, J.A.; Neuerer, F.; Hartmann, K.; Unterer, S. Effect of Amoxicillin-Clavulanic Acid on Clinical Scores, Intestinal Microbiome, and Amoxicillin-Resistant *Escherichia coli* in Dogs with Uncomplicated Acute Diarrhea. *J. Vet. Intern. Med.* **2020**, *34*, 1166–1176. [CrossRef] [PubMed]
34. Jakobsson, H.E.; Jernberg, C.; Andersson, A.F.; Sjölund-Karlsson, M.; Jansson, J.K.; Engstrand, L. Short-Term Antibiotic Treatment Has Differing Long-Term Impacts on the Human Throat and Gut Microbiome. *PLoS ONE* **2010**, *5*, e9836. [CrossRef] [PubMed]
35. Jernberg, C.; Löfmark, S.; Edlund, C.; Jansson, J.K. Long-Term Impacts of Antibiotic Exposure on the Human Intestinal Microbiota. *Microbiology* **2010**, *156*, 3216–3223. [CrossRef]
36. Rzewuska, M.; Czopowicz, M.; Kizerwetter-Świda, M.; Chrobak, D.; Błaszczak, B.; Binek, M. Multidrug Resistance in *Escherichia coli* Strains Isolated from Infections in Dogs and Cats in Poland (2007–2013). Available online: https://www.hindawi.com/journals/tswj/2015/408205/ (accessed on 9 October 2020). [CrossRef]
37. Escher, M.; Vanni, M.; Intorre, L.; Caprioli, A.; Tognetti, R.; Scavia, G. Use of Antimicrobials in Companion Animal Practice: A Retrospective Study in a Veterinary Teaching Hospital in Italy. *J. Antimicrob. Chemother.* **2011**, *66*, 920–927. [CrossRef]
38. Thomson, K.H.; Rantala, M.H.J.; Viita-Aho, T.K.; Vainio, O.M.; Kaartinen, L.A. Condition-Based Use of Antimicrobials in Cats in Finland: Results from Two Surveys. *J. Feline Med. Surg.* **2009**, *11*, 462–466. [CrossRef] [PubMed]
39. Odensvik, K.; Grave, K.; Greko, C. Antibacterial Drugs Prescribed for Dogs and Cats in Sweden and Norway 1990–1998. *Acta Vet. Scand.* **2001**, *42*, 189. [CrossRef] [PubMed]
40. Kvaale, M.K.; Grave, K.; Kristoffersen, A.B.; Norström, M. The Prescription Rate of Antibacterial Agents in Dogs in Norway—Geographical Patterns and Trends during the Period 2004–2008. *J. Vet. Pharmacol. Ther.* **2013**, *36*, 285–291. [CrossRef]
41. Mateus, A.; Brodbelt, D.C.; Barber, N.; Stärk, K.D.C. Antimicrobial Usage in Dogs and Cats in First Opinion Veterinary Practices in the UK. *J. Small Anim. Pract.* **2011**, *52*, 515–521. [CrossRef]
42. Marques, C.; Gama, L.T.; Belas, A.; Bergström, K.; Beurlet, S.; Briend-Marchal, A.; Broens, E.M.; Costa, M.; Criel, D.; Damborg, P.; et al. European Multicenter Study on Antimicrobial Resistance in Bacteria Isolated from Companion Animal Urinary Tract Infections. *BMC Vet. Res.* **2016**, *12*, 213. [CrossRef]
43. Joosten, P.; Ceccarelli, D.; Odent, E.; Sarrazin, S.; Graveland, H.; Van Gompel, L.; Battisti, A.; Caprioli, A.; Franco, A.; Wagenaar, J.A.; et al. Antimicrobial Usage and Resistance in Companion Animals: A Cross-Sectional Study in Three European Countries. *Antibiotics* **2020**, *9*, 87. [CrossRef]
44. Zhang, X.-F.; Doi, Y.; Huang, X.; Li, H.-Y.; Zhong, L.-L.; Zeng, K.-J.; Zhang, Y.-F.; Patil, S.; Tian, G.-B. Possible Transmission of *Mcr-1*–Harboring *Escherichia coli* between Companion Animals and Human. *Emerg. Infect. Dis.* **2016**, *22*, 1679–1681. [CrossRef]
45. Guenther, S.; Falgenhauer, L.; Semmler, T.; Imirzalioglu, C.; Chakraborty, T.; Roesler, U.; Roschanski, N. Environmental Emission of Multiresistant *Escherichia coli* Carrying the Colistin Resistance Gene *Mcr-1* from German Swine Farms. *J. Antimicrob. Chemother.* **2017**, dkw585. [CrossRef]
46. Comms, V. Colistin Resistance Detected in Shelter Dogs Imported from Russia. Available online: https://www.helsinki.fi/en/news/health/colistin-resistance-detected-in-shelter-dogs-imported-from-russia (accessed on 14 October 2020).
47. Ortega-Paredes, D.; Haro, M.; Leoro-Garzón, P.; Barba, P.; Loaiza, K.; Mora, F.; Fors, M.; Vinueza-Burgos, C.; Fernández-Moreira, E. Multidrug-Resistant *Escherichia coli* Isolated from Canine Faeces in a Public Park in Quito, Ecuador. *J. Glob. Antimicrob. Resist.* **2019**, *18*, 263–268. [CrossRef]
48. Grossman, T.H. Tetracycline Antibiotics and Resistance. *Cold Spring Harb. Perspect. Med.* **2016**, *6*, a025387. [CrossRef] [PubMed]
49. Chopra, I.; Roberts, M. Tetracycline Antibiotics: Mode of Action, Applications, Molecular Biology, and Epidemiology of Bacterial Resistance. *Microbiol. Mol. Biol. Rev.* **2001**, *65*, 232–260. [CrossRef]
50. Costa, D.; Poeta, P.; Sáenz, Y.; Coelho, A.C.; Matos, M.; Vinué, L.; Rodrigues, J.; Torres, C. Prevalence of Antimicrobial Resistance and Resistance Genes in Faecal *Escherichia coli* Isolates Recovered from Healthy Pets. *Vet. Microbiol.* **2008**, *127*, 97–105. [CrossRef] [PubMed]
51. Torkan, S.; Bahadoranian, M.; Khamesipour, F.; Anyanwu, M. Detection of Virulence and Antimicrobial Resistance Genes in *Escherichia coli* Isolates from Diarrhoiec Dogs in Iran. *Arch. Med. Vet.* **2016**, *48*, 181–190. [CrossRef]

52. Yousefi, A.; Torkan, S. Uropathogenic *Escherichia coli* in the Urine Samples of Iranian Dogs: Antimicrobial Resistance Pattern and Distribution of Antibiotic Resistance Genes. *BioMed Res. Int.* **2017**, *2017*, 1–10. [CrossRef]
53. Martinez-Martinez, L. Interaction of Plasmid and Host Quinolone Resistance. *J. Antimicrob. Chemother.* **2003**, *51*, 1037–1039. [CrossRef]
54. Yu, T.; Jiang, X.; Fu, K.; Liu, B.; Xu, D.; Ji, S.; Zhou, L. Detection of Extended-Spectrum β-Lactamase and Plasmid-Mediated Quinolone Resistance Determinants in *Escherichia coli* Isolates from Retail Meat in China: ESBL and PMQR Genes in *Escherichia coli*. *J. Food Sci.* **2015**, *80*, M1039–M1043. [CrossRef]
55. Ishida, Y.; Ahmed, A.M.; Mahfouz, N.B.; Kimura, T.; El-Khodery, S.A.; Moawad, A.A.; Shimamoto, T. Molecular Analysis of Antimicrobial Resistance in Gram-Negative Bacteria Isolated from Fish Farms in Egypt. *J. Vet. Med. Sci.* **2010**, *72*, 727–734. [CrossRef]
56. Zhao, X.; Xu, X.; Zhu, D.; Ye, X.; Wang, M. Decreased Quinolone Susceptibility in High Percentage of Enterobacter Cloacae Clinical Isolates Caused Only by Qnr Determinants. *Diagn. Microbiol. Infect. Dis.* **2010**, *67*, 110–113. [CrossRef]
57. Aslantas, Ö.; Yilmaz, E.S. Prevalence and Molecular Characterization of Extended-Spectrum β-Lactamase (ESBL) and Plasmidic AmpC β-Lactamase (PAmpC) Producing *Escherichia coli* in Dogs. *J. Vet. Med. Sci.* **2017**, *79*, 1024–1030. [CrossRef] [PubMed]
58. LeCuyer, T.E.; Byrne, B.A.; Daniels, J.B.; Diaz-Campos, D.V.; Hammac, G.K.; Miller, C.B.; Besser, T.E.; Davis, M.A. Population Structure and Antimicrobial Resistance of Canine Uropathogenic *Escherichia coli*. *J. Clin. Microbiol.* **2018**, *56*, e00788-18. [CrossRef]
59. Carvalho, A.C.; Barbosa, A.V.; Arais, L.R.; Ribeiro, P.F.; Carneiro, V.C.; Cerqueira, A.M.F. Resistance Patterns, ESBL Genes, and Genetic Relatedness of *Escherichia coli* from Dogs and Owners. *Braz. J. Microbiol.* **2016**, *47*, 150–158. [CrossRef] [PubMed]
60. Tenaillon, O.; Skurnik, D.; Picard, B.; Denamur, E. The Population Genetics of Commensal *Escherichia coli*. *Nat. Rev. Microbiol.* **2010**, *8*, 207–217. [CrossRef]
61. Russo, T.A.; Johnson, J.R. Proposal for a New Inclusive Designation for Extraintestinal Pathogenic Isolates of *Escherichia coli*: ExPEC. *J. Infect. Dis.* **2000**, *181*, 1753–1754. [CrossRef] [PubMed]
62. Hutton, T.A.; Innes, G.K.; Harel, J.; Garneau, P.; Cucchiara, A.; Schifferli, D.M.; Rankin, S.C. Phylogroup and Virulence Gene Association with Clinical Characteristics of *Escherichia coli* Urinary Tract Infections from Dogs and Cats. *J. Vet. Diagn. Investig.* **2018**, *30*, 64–70. [CrossRef]
63. Vega-Manriquez, X.D.; Ubiarco-López, A.; Verdugo-Rodríguez, A.; Hernández-Chiñas, U.; Navarro-Ocaña, A.; Ahumada-Cota, R.E.; Ramírez-Badillo, D.; Hernández-Díaz de León, N.; Eslava, C.A. Pet Dogs Potential Transmitters of Pathogenic *Escherichia coli* with Resistance to Antimicrobials. *Arch. Microbiol.* **2020**, *202*, 1173–1179. [CrossRef]
64. Valat, C.; Drapeau, A.; Beurlet, S.; Bachy, V.; Boulouis, H.-J.; Pin, R.; Cazeau, G.; Madec, J.-Y.; Haenni, M. Pathogenic *Escherichia coli* in Dogs Reveals the Predominance of ST372 and the Human-Associated ST73 Extra-Intestinal Lineages. *Front. Microbiol.* **2020**, *11*. [CrossRef]
65. Vijay, D.; Dhaka, P.; Vergis, J.; Negi, M.; Mohan, V.; Kumar, M.; Doijad, S.; Poharkar, K.; Kumar, A.; Malik, S.S.; et al. Characterization and Biofilm Forming Ability of Diarrhoeagenic Enteroaggregative *Escherichia coli* Isolates Recovered from Human Infants and Young Animals. *Comp. Immunol. Microbiol. Infect. Dis.* **2015**, *38*, 21–31. [CrossRef] [PubMed]
66. Tokuda, K.; Nishi, J.; Imuta, N.; Fujiyama, R.; Kamenosono, A.; Manago, K.; Kawano, Y. Characterization of Typical and Atypical Enteroaggregative *Escherichia coli* in Kagoshima, Japan: Biofilm Formation and Acid Resistance. *Microbiol. Immunol.* **2010**, *54*, 320–329. [CrossRef] [PubMed]
67. Navarro-Garcia, F.; Gutierrez-Jimenez, J.; Garcia-Tovar, C.; Castro, L.A.; Salazar-Gonzalez, H.; Cordova, V. Pic, an Autotransporter Protein Secreted by Different Pathogens in the Enterobacteriaceae Family, Is a Potent Mucus Secretagogue. *Infect. Immun.* **2010**, *78*, 4101–4109. [CrossRef] [PubMed]

MDPI
St. Alban-Anlage 66
4052 Basel
Switzerland
Tel. +41 61 683 77 34
Fax +41 61 302 89 18
www.mdpi.com

Microorganisms Editorial Office
E-mail: microorganisms@mdpi.com
www.mdpi.com/journal/microorganisms

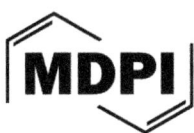

www.ingramcontent.com/pod-product-compliance
Lightning Source LLC
LaVergne TN
LVHW070556100526
838202LV00012B/485

9 7 8 3 0 3 6 5 2 7 8 1 9